the Macrobiotic

THE COMPLETE MACROBIOTIC DIET & EXERCISE BOOK

Other Avery books about macrobiotics:

The Changing Seasons Macrobiotic Cookbook
Cooking in Harmony with Nature
By Aveline Kushi and Wendy Esko

Lessons of Night and Day
Looking at the Balance of Nature
An illustrated children's book
By Aveline Kushi

The Macrobiotic Approach to Cancer
Towards Preventing & Controlling Cancer with Diet and Lifestyle
By Michio Kushi and the East West Foundation

On the Greater Life
Collected Thoughts and Ideas of Michio Kushi on Macrobiotics and
    Humanity

Shopper's Guide to Natural Foods
From the Editors of East West Journal

The Whole World Cookbook
International Macrobiotic Cuisine
From the Editors of East West Journal

Your Face Never Lies
An Introduction to Oriental Diagnosis
By Michio Kushi

the Macrobiotic Way

THE COMPLETE MACROBIOTIC DIET & EXERCISE BOOK

SECOND EDITION

MICHIO KUSHI
with Stephen Blauer

FOREWORD BY JOHN DENVER

AVERY PUBLISHING GROUP INC.
Garden City Park, New York

The health procedures in this book are based on the training, personal experiences, and research of the author. Because each person and situation is unique, the editor and publisher urge the reader to check with a qualified health professional before using any procedure where there is any question as to its appropriateness.

The publisher does not advocate the use of any particular diet and exercise program, but believes that the information presented in this book should be available to the public. If you have a history of back troubles or other physical restrictions, we recommend that you consult with your health care provider before beginning any exercise program.

Because there is always some risk involved, the author and publisher are not responsible for any adverse effects or consequences resulting from the use of any of the suggestions, preparations, or procedures in this book. Please do not use the book if you are unwilling to assume the risk. Feel free to consult a physician or other qualified health professional. It is a sign of wisdom, not cowardice, to seek a second or third opinion.

Cover design: Ann Vestal
Cover photograph: Pat Suth
Cover food stylist: Ann Vestal
In-house editor: Diana Puglisi
Printer: Paragon Press, Honesdale, PA

Library of Congress Cataloging-in-Publications Data

Kushi, Michio.
    The macrobiotic way.
    Includes index.
    1. Macrobiotic diet. 2. Exercise. 3. Health.
I. Blauer, Stephen. II. Title.
RM235.K873   1993   613.2'6 85-1324
ISBN 0-89529-524-5

Printed in the United States of America

10 9 8 7

Contents

Dedication

I dedicate this work to my wife, Aveline, and to my wonderful children. Further, I want to thank George and Lima Ohsawa, and the millions of people worldwide who share our dream of world peace, and happiness for everyone.

Preface

The earliest recorded use of the term macrobiotics is found in the writings of Hippocrates, the father of Western Medicine. In his essay "Airs, Waters, and Places," Hippocrates introduced the word to describe people who were healthy and long-lived. Translated from the Greek, "macro" means "large" or "great," and "bios" signifies "life." Herodotus, Aristotle, Galen, and other classical writers used the term macrobiotics to describe a lifestyle, including a simple balanced diet, that promoted health and longevity.

In the late eighteenth century, the German physician and philosopher Christophe W. Hufeland renewed interest in the term. His influential book on diet and health was entitled *Macrobiotics, or The Art of Prolonging Life.*

Nearly a century later, the term macrobiotics experienced a revival, this time originating in Japan. Two educators, Sagen Ishitsuka, M.D., and Yukikazu Sakurazawa, cured themselves of serious illnesses by adopting a simple diet of brown rice, miso soup, sea vegetables, and other traditional foods. These educators spent many years studying and integrating traditional Oriental medicine and Eastern philosophy with Judeo-Christian teachings and wholistic perspectives in modern science and medicine. Sakurazawa came to Paris in the 1920s. Later he adopted the name George Ohsawa, and applied the term macrobiotics to his teachings.

From the time of his illness until his death at the age of seventy-four, Ohsawa devoted himself to defining macrobiotics as it applies to modern living. He did much to spread information about the macrobiotic lifestyle, visiting more than thirty countries, giving more than seven thousand lectures, and publishing over three hundred books.

Ohsawa had many students, among them Michio Kushi, the author of this book. Kushi was born in 1926 and graduated from Tokyo University with a degree in international law before coming to the United States in 1949. While completing further studies at Columbia University in New York, he also began teaching the macrobiotic approach to diet and health. Kushi enjoyed sharing his knowledge of macrobiotics and natural health with others so much that he made it his life's work.

When Kushi began teaching macrobiotics, he met many people who were eager to learn, but were unaccustomed to eating simple whole foods. He saw that there was a need to adapt the macrobiotic diet to modern tastes, while retaining its integrity. Over the years, Kushi has traveled extensively, lecturing and teaching the macrobiotic way to groups around the world. He and his associates are frequently invited to speak at the United Nations in New York, where a macrobiotic association has been formed.

Macrobiotics advocates the use of traditional foods such as whole grains, beans, and locally grown vegetables as primary sources of food energy and nutrition. In addition, the diet includes nutritious soyfoods, which have been used in the Orient for hundreds of years, and mineral-rich foods from the ocean—sea vegetables and certain types of fish. On the macrobiotic diet, moderate amounts of white-meat fish and shellfish are often substituted for red meat and poultry. Sea salt and natural grain sweeteners such as rice syrup and barley malt replace the refined salt and sugar that currently play a major role in modern fare.

When Michio Kushi first accepted the challenge of helping people shift to a more healthful way of eating and living, he had trouble finding many of the wholesome foods that he recommended. So, with his wife Aveline, he started a natural foods business to fill the need. Later to be called Erewhon, this small enterprise developed into a $17 million business specializing in macrobiotic and natural foods.

To research and popularize the macrobiotic approach, Michio and Aveline Kushi have founded the East West Foundation and the Kushi Institute, both non-profit educational organizations; the *East West Journal*, a monthly magazine that currently has a world-wide circulation of over seventy-five thousand; and several macrobiotic restaurants. The Kushis have five children and five grandchildren.

Michio and Aveline Kushi have written many books on macrobiotics, including *The Book of Macrobiotics; The Book of Do-In: Exercise for Physical and Spiritual Development; The Cancer Prevention Diet; Your Face Never Lies: An Introduction to Oriental Diagnosis; The Macrobiotic Approach to Cancer; Natural Healing Through Macrobiotics; How to Cook with Miso; The Changing Seasons Macrobiotic Cookbook,* and *Macrobiotic Pregnancy and Care of the Newborn.* Michio Kushi is also the author of a series of books, *Teachings of Michio Kushi.*

During the last two years I have come to know Michio and Aveline Kushi well. They are extraordinary people with endless reserves of energy, patience, and compassion for others. As a scholar, philosopher, writer, and teacher, Michio Kushi is often busy from early in the morning until after midnight. Whether he is greeting individuals for counseling sessions, discussing plans for the further development and growth of the macrobiotic way, attending a session of the macrobiotic scientific committee, giving a seminar for medical and health care professionals, or just talking about life with a friend, Kushi is always actively sharing his boundless enthusiasm for living and his ability to view life's problems with gentle good humor.

This book is the result of my desire to understand Michio Kushi's macrobiotic approach to diet and health and to explain it in simple terms to a general audience. Michio Kushi is the author of this book inasmuch as its contents are derived from discussions with him. In addition, material from his lectures, published books, and articles, has been drawn upon.

Both Michio and I are indebted to our families and friends for their valuable assistance in preparing this book. We would especially like to thank Aveline Kushi and Wendy Esko for helping to develop the recipes and cooking sections, with the assistance of Karen Williamson, Caroline Heindenry, and Colleen Blauer. Special thanks also go to Lawrence Haruo Kushi of the Harvard School of Public Health, to Phillip Kushi and Ed Esko of the East West Foundation, to Bill Tara of the Kushi Institute, and to Lenny Jacobs, Linda Roszak, and Mark Mayell of the *East West Journal,* for reviewing the style, tone, accuracy, and clarity of the other sections of the book.

We are also grateful to our editor at Avery Publishing Group, Diana Puglisi, whose editorial excellence, and patience, helped make our manuscript into a book. In addition, we would like to thank Lydia Wilen for her literary assistance and support. Above all, we extend special thanks to the Managing Editor of Avery Publishing Group, Rudy Shur, for his encouragement, enthusiasm, and assistance throughout.

My greatest hope is that the spirit of sharing and cooperation, through which this book became a reality, will somehow touch the lives of its readers. For in giving is to be found abundance, peace, and happiness.

Stephen Blauer
Boston, Massachusetts

Foreword

A few years ago, as I was preparing a major concert tour in the United States, I realized that I wanted to have someone to cook for me and help me to keep my body in good shape while on the road. I was beginning to eat less and less red meat and sugar, and knew then I wanted to pursue a "vegetarian" diet. (Albeit, I was and still am a chocoholic, and was a great admirer of ice cream.) Lo and behold, a man named Ron Lemire, who was an expert (professional) cook and masseur, appeared and offered to take on the job. In the following months, I did 125 concerts in 100 cities across the country. The general procedure was to be out on the road for two weeks, then at home for two weeks. While on the road and eating Ron's food, I had incredible energy, great clarity of mind and inner peace (a lack of susceptibility to stress and pressure). My voice was stronger and clearer than it had ever been, and I felt light and good and healthy.

At home, following my normal diet, I felt quite different. The food was very rich, lots of sauces and spices, and sugar and cream. To be honest, my discipline at home is not what it is on the road, and I could not keep my hands out of the cookie jar or stay away from the ice cream in the refrigerator. In reality, I didn't sleep well, felt quite lethargic and stiff, and was more prone to anger or upset—basically, I didn't feel good.

Now my Dad and Mom didn't raise any stupid children. After about five mini-tours, I realized that the only difference in my life on the road and at home was the food I was eating. Also, I began to notice that there was a pattern or form to the food Ron was giving me on the road. My main meal in the middle of the day consisted of a soup, a grain, some beans, some steamed vegetables, a salad and a great dessert. It didn't seem to be "just vegetarian." There was a discipline involved. I then began to learn about the Macrobiotic Way; about yin and yang, about balance and about Michio Kushi and his good work.

Since that time I have had the privilege of getting to know Michio and Aveline, their family and friends in Brookline, Massachusetts, and other macrobiotic friends at East West centers all over the world. I have had the opportunity to play a small part in their ongoing work to bring about a more healthy and happy life for all people and to create a world of peace.

In the process, my own feelings of a human family have been strengthened and clarified. As my knowledge of diet and health increases, so does my conviction. We can end hunger on this planet. We can cure cancer and heart disease. Peace is possible.

No one is working more energetically or effectively toward those ends than Michio Kushi and his family and friends—all those who follow the Macrobiotic Way.

Peace,
John Denver
Aspen, Colorado

Introduction

Macrobiotics is a way of eating and living that has been practiced for thousands of years by many people around the world. It stems from an intuitive understanding of the orderliness of nature. Modern macrobiotic philosophy focuses on offering a way of living that closes the widening gap between humans and the natural world. Macrobiotic theory suggests that sickness and unhappiness are nature's way of urging us to adopt a proper diet and way of life, and that these troubles are unnecessary when we live in harmony with our environment. The macrobiotic diet is based on whole grains and traditional foods in harmony with the seasons.

As we have become somewhat removed from the natural elements, we have lost much that is valuable. We can learn a great deal from peoples such as the Hunzakuts, Vilcabambans, and Abkhasians, who often live in continuous close contact with nature. They are vitally healthy and very active physically, many beyond their one-hundredth birthday. Most of the foods they eat are locally and organically grown, vegetarian, and unprocessed. Their diet is essentially macrobiotic, as it is based primarily on whole cereal grains such as wheat, barley, buckwheat, corn, and brown rice, with fresh vegetables and greens, peas, nuts, beans, and fruits. Though they do eat some meat, dairy products, and poultry, these constitute less than one percent of their diet.

We may not be able to adopt these peoples' level of activity (although many people feel we should), or their more rustic lifestyle, but we can adopt a more wholesome diet. In fact, recent nutritional research performed for the United States government recommends a more simple approach to diet. Two publications, *Dietary Goals for the United States* (1977), and *Diet, Nutrition and Cancer* (1982), have come out in favor of sweeping dietary changes, including more whole grains, whole grain products, beans, fresh vegetables, and fruits, and fewer red meats, cheeses, eggs, poultry, and highly refined foods lacking fiber. The studies also recommend reducing salt, sugar, and fat consumption.

The hundreds of medical and nutritional scientists who contributed to the government reports believe the dietary changes they suggest can reduce the incidence of heart disease, hypertension, obesity, gall bladder and liver disorders, and cancer. The first report, issued by the McGovern Senate Select Committee on Nutrition and Human Needs, concluded that our present eating habits "may be as profoundly damaging to the nation's health as the widespread contagious diseases of the early part of the century."

Although these monumental studies received little, if any, attention from the news media, thousands of people are turning to alternatives such as the macrobiotic diet to prevent illness and improve health. Several well-known physicians, including Dr. Keith Block, a medical/nutritional consultant for CBS radio in Chicago, and Dr. Robert Mendelsohn, former medical director of the American International Hospital in Zion, Illinois, praise the macrobiotic diet as a ray of hope in the prevention of illness.

Drs. Edward Kass and Frank Sacks of Harvard University reported in the *American Journal of Epidemology*, May, 1974, that the macrobiotic diet normalized blood pressure. Their study of 210 individuals who switched to macrobiotics showed that the largely vegetarian diet was effective in bringing high blood pressure down to normal levels, and maintained these levels far more effectively than the diet eaten by the average American.

A year later, the *New England Journal of Medicine* published another study by Drs. Kass and Sacks, this time stating that people who switched to the macrobiotic diet had healthier-than-average blood fat and cholesterol levels, despite having eaten the typical modern diet (which tends to elevate blood fat and cholesterol levels) most of their lives. In 1982, J.T. Knuiman and C.E. West confirmed Dr. Kass's findings in their own research, which compared the total blood fat and cholesterol levels of macrobiotic, vegetarian, and non-vegetarian males. Their report was published in the journal *Atherosclerosis*.

The success of the macrobiotic diet in controlling blood pressure, fat, and cholesterol levels has made it medically credible. Some physicians are now recommending it to their patients along with standard treatment. In fact, at Boston's Lemuel Shattuck general hospital, wholesome macrobiotic meals are available to the staff and some patients. In Linho, Portugal, a group of prisoners have been given the opportunity to eat macrobiotically. Chico Varatojo, director of a macrobiotic center for the prison, feels that the poorly balanced nutrition of the conventional diet is largely responsible for crime and delinquency in modern society.

It is best to adopt the macrobiotic diet with a confident and unhurried attitude. Begin by adding whole foods such as pressure-cooked brown rice to your present diet, and gradually increase the variety of natural foods and cooking styles you use. Eliminate strong-tasting spices and seasonings, and replace them with appropriate cooking methods that enable the inherent flavor and vitality of natural foods to come through. With the help of the chapters on food preparation and the recipes in this book, you will be well on the way to preparing delectable macrobiotic meals as if you have been doing so all your life. You may also want to attend macrobiotic cooking classes, which are offered in many parts of the United States (see Appendix E).

Unlike most other diets, macrobiotics has continued to grow and expand its sphere of influence for over fifty years. Macrobiotic educators have been pioneers of the natural and organic foods revolution. Today there are more than five hundred learning centers teaching macrobiotics worldwide. In just about any large city, from Dublin to Dallas and from Athens to Atlanta, you will find people following the macrobiotic way. In many cities you will find one or more macrobiotic restaurants, or restaurants that serve macrobiotic meals. At the Fenway Howard Johnson's motor lodge in Boston, for example, guests can enjoy a complete macrobiotic breakfast.

Throughout this book you will read about individuals who, after suffering with poor health for a time, tried macrobiotics and discovered that it truly helped them. In all of the cases, three factors contributed to successful recovery: the proper quality, quantity, and combination of well-prepared food; regular exercise; and a positive mental outlook. These aspects of the macrobiotic way are the focal points of this book.

In Chapter 1 you will learn what the macrobiotic diet consists of, how it compares to the diet currently eaten in many parts of the world, and how you can use macrobiotics to improve your health and that of your family.

HOWARD Johnson's *motor lodge*

The Flavor of America

1271 BOYLSTON STREET
BOSTON, MASSACHUSETTS 02215
(617) 267-8300

Dear Macrobiotic Guest:

We at the Howard Johnson's are delighted to announce our new addition to the Bumper's Breakfast Menu - our special Macrobiotic Breakfast!! Our restaurant staff has been trained in the proper preparation of these foods and will serve them with our guest's best interest in mind.

BUMPER'S

Macrobiotic Breakfast Menu

Bowl of Rolled Oats..............................$1.00

All Natural Whole Wheat Toast

        Plain..............................$ .75

        With Sesame Butter..............$1.10

        With Apple Butter...............$1.10

Cup of Instant Miso Soup.....................$1.25

Pure Unsweetened Apple Cider

        Small.............................$1.00

        Large.............................$1.25

Bancha Tea...................................$ .60

Condiments Include:
Toasted Sesame Salt
&
Barley Malt Sweetener

Reprinted by permission of Howard Johnson's Fenway Motor Lodge, Boston, MA. Copyright 1984.

1

The Way to Better Health

The macrobiotic approach to diet, exercise, and living can lead to better health for you and your family. If you choose to eat macrobiotically, and follow the other suggestions in this book, you will reap the rewards of an active, intelligent, energizing approach to life. You will discover richness and harmony in nature, even amidst the pressures and hazards of our complicated world.

Macrobiotic philosophy teaches that a wholesome diet is the most direct path to good health, so the first part of this book is directed to examining the role of nutrition in the macrobiotic way. More so than any other approach to diet, macrobiotics appreciates and emphasizes individual differences such as where you live, what you do, and your present state of health.

Based on the philosophic principles of balance and harmony, the idea behind the diet is simple: your climate or geographical location, activity level, and physiology determine your nutritional needs. In making dietary choices, these factors are far better guides to follow than general nutritional and caloric tables.

In addition, macrobiotics points out the harmful effect modern methods of food processing and refining have upon our physical and mental health. The macrobiotic diet uses only whole foods and foods that are processed by traditional methods.

WHOLE, UNPROCESSED FOODS

Unlike the people of Hunza, Vilcabamba, and other traditional cultures, who eat locally grown whole grains, fresh vegetables, and fruits, with few (if any) processed foods containing chemical ad-

1

ditives, Americans have come to rely primarily on processed foods. Alex Schauss, in *Diet, Crime, and Delinquency*, notes: "In 1971, the U.S. had the dubious distinction of becoming the first nation on earth to consume processed foods for more than 50 percent of its diet." Samuel Epstein, M.D., in *The Politics of Cancer*, tells us that the average American now consumes nine pounds of chemical additives per year, in the form of preservatives, artificial colorings and flavorings, and texture agents. This "American" diet is actually fairly typical of the average diet in other affluent industrialized nations as well. Yet, as the longevity and general good health of people whose diets contain few processed foods attest, the use of chemical food additives is not necessary for the maintenance of good health.

An excess of calories and saturated animal fats, coupled with nutrient loss in processing and the use of additives, is largely responsible for the staggering rate of health problems in many Western nations. The National Center for Health Statistics report *Current Health Interviews Survey* states that nearly one in every two Americans has a chronic condition that may result in disease of some sort. To reverse this situation, the macrobiotic diet recommends eating whole foods, primarily of plant origin, which are lower in calories, contain less saturated fat and no chemical additives, and require little or no processing.

LOCALLY GROWN FOODS

Each region of the United States (and of the world), through its geography and climate, places certain demands and stresses on the people who live there. Eating foods which are grown in the same conditions as those in which we live enables us to adapt more successfully to the changes taking place around us. A person living in a cold, wet climate such as Scotland or Ireland would do well to eat the oil-rich oats that have traditionally been consumed there. Someone living in the southern United States, on the other hand, would be better off eating brown rice or the sweeter corn products grown in that region.

As much of our food as possible should be native to the area in which we live. For a New Englander to eat Florida oranges or Costa

Rican bananas is to ignore the close connection between the body and its immediate environment, thus inviting seasonal imbalances such as colds and flu, and possibly more serious illness.

Most residents of the United States live in the temperate zone, north of the Tropic of Cancer and south of the Arctic Circle. The foods that grow naturally in the temperate zone—especially whole grains, beans, seeds, vegetables, and some fruits—are balanced nutritionally for those of us who live where they are grown and harvested.

THE MACROBIOTIC DIET IN PERSPECTIVE

A comparison of the macrobiotic diet with the one eaten in modernized societies and the one recommended by a government panel in the publication *Dietary Goals For the United States*, is illustrated on the following page.

The macrobiotic diet is comprised of whole foods. Most of the food energy comes from complex carbohydrates. On the macrobiotic diet, proper cooking methods preserve nutrients and enhance flavor in foods. Highly processed foods containing additives, commercial salt, and cane or beet sugar are avoided as much as possible. Dairy products, red meat, poultry, and foods containing these ingredients are generally not recommended for people living in temperate climates.

The *Dietary Goals* recommendations do not exclude heavily processed food items containing additives and preservatives. This diet is still too high in saturated fats, cholesterol, and highly refined vegetable fats to be considered optimally healthful. No special recommendations are made on cooking procedures or on balancing the diet. Yet, these recommendations are a tremendous improvement over the way most of us eat now.

The modern diet relies heavily on processed and synthetic foods. It is much too high in saturated animal fats, cholesterol, and highly refined vegetable fats, and it is deficient in complex carbohydrates, fiber, and natural vitamins and minerals. Excessively high in salt, sugar, and chemical additives (some 3,500 have found their way into our food supply), the modern diet is increasingly subject to criticism from a standpoint of nutritional quantity and quality.

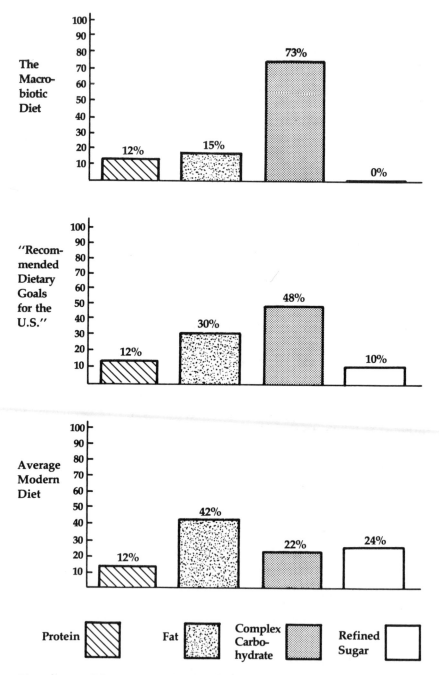

Figure 1.1   Three-Way Comparison

THE STANDARD MACROBIOTIC DIET

The macrobiotic diet consists of: 50–60 percent whole grains and whole grain products; 20–30 percent locally grown (when possible, organically grown) vegetables; 5–10 percent beans and sea vegetables; 5–10 percent soups; and 5 percent condiments and supplementary foods, including beverages, fish, and desserts. Figure 1.2 shows the proportions of the diet in graphic form.

Many of the foods that form an important part of the standard macrobiotic diet may be unfamiliar to you. These foods, and the menu mentioned below, will become more meaningful as you read this book and sample the recipes. On the macrobiotic diet, you can look forward to delicious and healthful eating as a way of life. If you would like to find out more about macrobiotic foods right away, turn to the Glossary on page 219.

Although red meats, poultry, dairy products, and foods prepared with them are generally not recommended for people in temperate

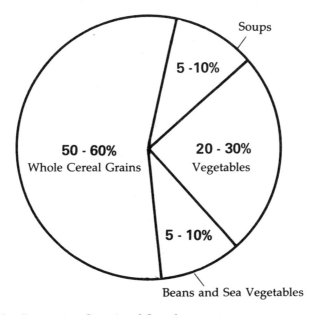

Plus Beverages, Occasional Supplementary
Foods, Seasonings, and Condiments

Figure 1.2   General Proportions of the Macrobiotic Diet

Breakfast
Oatmeal Whole Wheat Sourdough Toast with Apple Butter Bancha Tea
Lunch
Cucumber Sushi and Tempeh-Sauerkraut Sushi Boiled Salad with Tofu Dressing Bancha Tea with Lemon
Dinner
Miso Soup Baked Sole with Rice Grated Daikon with Toasted Nori Strips Quickly Boiled Watercress and Carrots with Umeboshi-Scallion Dressing Couscous Cake with Pear Sauce Grain Coffee
Snacks (optional)
Roasted seeds or nuts with raisins, rice balls, rice cakes, home-made popcorn, seasonal fruits (cooked, dried, or fresh), mochi cakes (made from sweet brown rice), unleavened whole wheat crackers.

climate zones, the macrobiotic diet need not be completely vegetarian. It includes small amounts of white-meat fish and certain shellfish. Richly nourishing tofu and tempeh (soy products which are minimally processed using traditional methods without chemicals), are used in place of other animal foods. Seitan, a protein-rich wheat product; amasake, a sweet milk-like drink made from brown rice; and a number of other supplementary foods we will discuss more fully later on, are also included in the diet, often in place of meat and dairy products.

Whole foods are eaten as close to their natural form as possible. In place of refined grains or flours we suggest you use brown rice with only the outer hull removed, whole oats, whole rye, whole wheat, corn, buckwheat, and millet. Flours made from whole wheat, rye, buckwheat, and corn can replace white flour for making breads and pasta. Whole grain breakfast cereals can be made from whole or rolled oats, freshly ground cornmeal, brown rice, and so on. A typical day's menu might look something like the one on page 6.

Denmark's "Macrobiotic Experiment"

During the First World War, Denmark was blockaded, and widespread food shortages and malnutrition were a very real threat. Mikkel Hinhede, superintendent of the Danish State Institute of Food Research, was appointed food advisor to the Danish government. Hinhede not only solved the problem—he achieved a complete reversal of the situation.

In the years before the war, Denmark imported inexpensive grain. Danish farmers bred pigs, cattle, and poultry, and sent eggs and butter to England. The Danes themselves were big eaters of meat and eggs. After the blockade, however, their grain supply was cut off, and there were over 5,000,000 grain-eating domestic animals and 3,500,000 people to feed.

Immediately, Hinhede ordered that four-fifths of the pigs and one-fifth of the cattle be killed, so that more grain would be available for human consumption. In addition, consumption of pork and other meats was reduced or eliminated altogether. Hinhede also limited the production of alcoholic beverages, knowing that the grain used to make them could be better used to make a special whole meal bread called *Kleiebrot*. The Danes began to eat more porridge, more fresh greens, vegetables, peas, beans, and fruits, and lesser amounts of milk and butter.

From October, 1917, to October, 1918, the most trying period of the war, Denmark became the healthiest nation in Europe. In one year on a diet similar to the macrobiotic diet, the cancer rate dropped by 60 percent and the death rate fell more than 40 percent. After the war, the Danes adopted their former diet and the mortality rate quickly returned to prewar levels. ■

From Mikkel Hinhede, "The Effects of Food Restriction During War on Mortality in Copenhagen," *Journal of the American Medical Association* 74 (1920): 381–382.

2
The Best Foods You Can Eat

Do you avoid starches because you have heard that they are fattening? You may be surprised to learn that the complex, natural starches found in whole grains such as brown rice or whole wheat, and in vegetables, are in reality the best foods we can eat. Natural foods, which contain complex carbohydrates, are energy foods. Compared with proteins or fats, complex carbohydrates provide the body with more easily usable fuel for energy, and leave behind fewer waste products.

Nearly everyone eats carbohydrates in some form at each meal. However, in our modern world, where processed and refined foods are readily available, up to half of the carbohydrates eaten by the average individual are supplied in the form of simple carbohydrates. The problem is that simple, refined carbohydrates can damage our health.

COMPLEX VERSUS SIMPLE CARBOHYDRATES

A doughnut and coffee with cream and sugar in the morning, and a candy bar in the afternoon, may seem to give you a lift, but in reality these simple carbohydrate foods cause fatigue within a few minutes, when the sugar leaves the bloodstream. What happens is that the insulin level shoots up to counteract the overly quick release of sugar. This brings the blood sugar level down, way down, so that you start feeling tense, and hungry for more sugar. Day after day, your body takes an uncomfortable roller coaster ride, and your emotions can't help rising and falling along with it.

The macrobiotic diet replaces simple carbohydrates with more complex, slower-burning ones. Brown rice, for example, releases a continuous stream of glucose into the blood at a rate of about two calories per minute. The sugar in a candy bar is burned more quickly, releasing thirty or more calories per minute. Simple sugars such as honey, refined white sugar, and even fruit sugars, are absorbed quickly because they are digested without the use of pancreatic enzymes, but they do not provide long-lasting energy. A macrobiotic meal of whole grains, vegetables, and beans will release its energy over a period of hours, without resulting in wide swings of mood or hunger for sweets.

ENERGY FOOD VERSUS BUILDING FOOD

Carbohydrates give us energy, whereas proteins help us to build and renew cells, muscles, and tissues. Even though the body contains a large amount of protein, our primary dietary need is for energy to maintain a balanced internal state. Carbohydrates must be supplied continuously in the diet because the body can only store small reserves of them. Only when the supply of carbohydrates is insufficient, as in starvation, does the body begin to break down proteins for energy.

The people of Hunza, well-known for their overall good health and longevity, get about 75 percent of their total caloric intake from complex carbohydrates, with the other 25 percent coming from proteins and fats. The ratio of complex carbohydrate to protein in their diet is about six or seven to one—identical to the macrobiotic diet. In contrast, the diet in many parts of the world contains about 12 percent protein and only 22 percent complex carbohydrates—about a two to one ratio (see Figure 1.1).

This means the average individual's body must work much harder, because it is forced to convert a portion of the fats and proteins consumed into energy. In addition, these conversions create waste products which must be acted upon by the liver and kidneys and eliminated from the body. The mainstays of the macrobiotic diet, on the other hand, are clean-burning complex carbohydrates that are converted by the body into glucose for energy, carbon dioxide that is exhaled, and water.

SWEET LOW, SWEET HIGH

The quality of the carbohydrates consumed is just as important as the quantity. A lack of complex carbohydrates, along with an excess of simple carbohydrates, is largely responsible for the problem of hypoglycemia (low blood sugar). Hypoglycemia first reveals itself as insatiable hunger, which may remain even on a full stomach. Fatigue, excessive perspiration, yawning, shaking, and uncontrollable emotions are a few of the other symptoms.

More than ten million Americans suffer from hypoglycemia, some of them without ever knowing it. At first glance this would appear to be an absurdity: how could so many people have low blood sugar while consuming an average of nearly two pounds of sugar a week? If you recall our discussion of simple carbohydrates, you can see how it is the sugar itself that causes the problem.

Since sugar, in the form of glucose, supplies energy to the whole body, a lack of it can weaken every organ, including the brain, which depends on sugar to function properly. When too much sugar is eaten, however, it actually reduces the amount of sugar available to the body for energy.

The islets of Langerhans are tiny glands, located in the pancreas, which are responsible for the production of the hormone insulin. They become overstimulated when there are excessive quantities of fast-burning sugar in the diet. For example, when a person with hypoglycemia consumes a candy bar or soft drink, the islets spurt insulin into the blood, lowering blood sugar levels and depleting stores of glycogen (a source of quick energy held in reserve in the liver). Unable to increase the blood sugar level without glycogen, the liver sends an SOS to the brain for help—and all of a sudden the hypoglycemic craves more sugar. If additional sugar is consumed, the cycle is repeated. If not, the body secretes the hormone adrenalin, which, among other things, makes sugar available for energy in emergencies. The release of adrenalin is in part responsible for the symptoms mentioned earlier. And even though a doctor may tell hypoglycemic patients not to eat sugar, many still do, because they do not understand why it is bad for them.

The standard recommendation for hypoglycemics is to follow a high-protein diet. In the short run, this seems to work fine. Every time patients feel a craving for sugar, they are instructed to eat a high-protein item to satisfy it. With a short supply of glycogen in the liver, the body is forced to convert protein into glucose for fuel. Making this conversion requires a tremendous amount of energy, and after a few weeks the hypoglycemic often finds it impossible to follow a high-protein regimen. Totally exhausted, and craving sweets more than ever, he or she goes off the diet.

Years of experience in working with hypoglycemics has led me to a different approach to the problem. Hypoglycemics need no more protein than anybody else. What they need most is the same thing we all need to have plenty of—fuel for energy, in the form of complex carbohydrates. It is best for those suffering from hypoglycemia to avoid sugar and refined foods. Moreover, hypoglycemics may need to eat smaller, more frequent meals for a time. This is a relatively simple transition once an individual decides to do it, because the absolutely safe form of sugar, slowly released by the macrobiotic diet, replaces lost energy and reduces the craving for sweets. Every situation and every individual is different, however. Questions regarding personal needs should be brought to a trained macrobiotic counselor (see Appendix E).

The Sweet Life of a Sugar Junkie

For years, my friend William Dufty, radio personality and author of Lady Sings The Blues, *loved to eat sugar. "I must have been hooked very early," he says, "because my earliest memories of mealtime at home with the family was a kind of purgatory of meat and potatoes which I suffered through in order to get to heaven: a sweet dessert."*

It wasn't until years later, though, while seated next to actress Gloria Swanson at a New York luncheon press conference, that Bill awoke to his problem. He was about to drop a sugar cube into his coffee when Gloria whispered, "That stuff is poison, I won't have it in my house, let alone my body." The conversation that followed stayed on his mind for days. He was overweight and felt lousy much of the time.

After Bill met Gloria and discovered macrobiotics, he gave up eating sugar and went on to write about his experiences. In the introduction to his book Sugar Blues, *he writes:*

. . . One night, in one sitting, I read a little book that said very simply if you're sick, it's your own fault. Pain is the final warning. You know better than anyone else how you've been abusing your body, so stop it. Sugar is poison, it said, more lethal than opium and more dangerous than atomic fallout. Shades of Gloria Swanson and the sugar cube. Hadn't she told me everyone has to find out themselves—the hard way? I had nothing to lose but my pains. I began the next morning with firm resolve. I threw all the sugar out of my kitchen. Then I threw out everything that had sugar in it, cereals and canned fruit, soups and bread. Since I had never read any labels carefully I was shocked to find the shelves were soon empty; so was the refrigerator. I began eating nothing but whole grains and vegetables. . .

. . . I had it very rough for about twenty-four hours, but the morning after was a revelation. I went to sleep with exhaustion, sweating and tremors. I woke up feeling reborn. Grains and vegetables tasted like a gift from the gods.

The next few days brought a succession of wonders. My rear stopped bleeding, so did my gums. My skin began to clear up and had a totally different texture when I washed. I discovered bones in my hands and feet that had been buried under bloat. I bounced out of bed at strange hours in the morning. My head seemed to be working again. I had no problems anymore. My shirts were too big. So were my shoes. One morning I discovered my jaw.

To make a long, happy story short, I dropped from 205 pounds to a neat 135 in five months and ended up with a new body, a new head, a new life. . . ■

Bill has been eating macrobiotically for years now, and still comes by often to see us in Brookline. He has conveyed to me privately that the "little book" that changed his life was Macrobiotics, *by George Ohsawa.*

Reprinted from *Sugar Blues,* © 1975 William Dufty. Used by Permission. Warner Books Edition currently in print.

3

Protein and the Macrobiotic Diet

Proteins are complex molecules found in almost all living things. Whereas carbohydrates are the best source of food energy, proteins are the best source of raw material for the vital processes of growth and repair.

Proteins are the building blocks of the human body. They are found abundantly in the muscles, tendons, blood, and organs. The hair, fingernails, and skin are all made of protein. Yet it is not protein itself that we need in our diet, but the components of proteins known as amino acids.

In the process of digestion, the body breaks down proteins into amino acids. The amino acids supplied by foods, along with those recycled internally, are reassembled by the liver, creating the proteins required by the body for the repair of cells and tissues, for growth, and to maintain metabolic processes. Of the twenty-two amino acids needed to maintain health, eight of them, known as the essential amino acids, can be obtained only from food. The body is able to manufacture the others from various substances.

This chapter considers protein and the macrobiotic diet from two perspectives: how the quality and quantity of protein in the diet affect health, particularly athletic performance; and how protein consumption relates to the problem of world hunger.

PROTEIN AND THE MACROBIOTIC DIET

The macrobiotic diet supplies protein, including the eight essential amino acids, from the best available protein sources—whole grains, beans, vegetables, sea vegetables, seeds, nuts, white-meat fish, and fruit. Other protein sources, such as red meat, poultry, and milk, generally contain a high percentage of substances which can contribute to coronary disease and other health problems.

Many people today eat far too much protein, and since foods that are high in protein are often high in fat, these people may be eating too much fat (especially too much saturated animal fat) as well. Excessive protein in the diet can result in accumulations of urea, uric acid, fat, and cholesterol in body tissues and in the blood. Excess acid and fat in the blood tend to wash away stores of essential minerals, such as iron, magnesium, zinc, phosphorus, and calcium, causing the bones and teeth to weaken. In addition, as the National Academy of Sciences publication *Diet, Nutrition, and Cancer*, suggests, high protein intake may increase the risk of cancer of the breast, colon, rectum, pancreas, prostate gland, and kidneys.

Table 3.1 summarizes the nutritional composition of various foods. The percentages for protein, fat, and carbohydrate are based on the total caloric value of the particular food. For example, in brown rice, 7% of the calories come from protein, 4% come from fat, and 89% come from carbohydrate. In the root vegetable daikon, 16% of the calories come from protein, 5% come from fat, and 80% come from carbohydrate.

On the average, about 12% of the total caloric intake on the macrobiotic diet comes from protein, 15% comes from fat, and 73% comes from complex carbohydrates. The way to achieve this ideal balance is to eat a variety of foods that offer an optimal amount of high-quality protein, without excessive amounts of saturated fats or cholesterol.

IF YOU'RE AN ATHLETE

The myths surrounding nutrition are at present only beginning to fade. Let us examine a few of them. It is commonly believed that in order to build up big, strong muscles you need lots of protein. This is simply not the case. Even a body-builder's need for protein is the same as anyone else's. It is prolonged, strenuous exercise, not protein, that builds and strengthens muscles.

Another common myth is that when you use your muscles vigorously in sports or exercise it causes them to deteriorate, so that extra protein is needed to rebuild them. But, as early as 1866, pioneering

Table 3.1   Percentages of Protein, Fat, and Carbohydrate

	% Protein	% Fat (unsaturated)	% Carbohydrate
Whole Grains and Whole Grain Products			
Barley, pearled	8	2	89
Brown rice	7	4	89
Buckwheat, noodles	12	6	82
Buckwheat, whole grain	12	6	82
Cornmeal, whole–ground	7	9	84
Millet, whole	3	8	70
Oatmeal	13	16	72
Popcorn	9	11	80
Rye	11	4	85
Wheat, bulghur	10	3	82
Wheat, noodles	9	3	84
Wheat, whole	5	13	81
Vegetables			
Bean sprouts	27	5	68
Broccoli	27	8	66
Brussels sprouts	28	9	63
Cabbage	13	7	80
Carrots	7	4	89
Cauliflower	24	6	69
Celery	13	5	82
Collard greens	23	17	60
Corn, sweet	9	9	81
Daikon	16	5	80
Kale	28	21	51
Lettuce, romaine	18	14	69
Mushrooms	25	9	55
Mustard greens	23	14	62
Onions	11	2	88
Parsley	20	11	69
Parsnips	6	6	87
Peas, green	26	5	69
Pumpkin	7	7	85
String beans	16	8	76
Squash, winter	7	5	88
Rutabagas	7	2	90
Turnips	10	7	83
Watercress	29	13	57

Table 3.1—*Continued*

	% Protein	% Fat (unsaturated)	% Carbohydrate
Beans			
Aduki beans	23	3	74
Black or brown beans	23	4	74
Chick peas	20	11	69
Lentils	26	trace	74
Lima beans	20	4	75
Pinto beans	23	3	74
Soybeans	29	37	34
Split peas	24	2	74

Source: Based on data from the United States Department of Agriculture Handbook No. 8, *Composition of Foods*, and from the Japan Nutritionist Association.

Note: One value is given for both cooked and raw foods, as the percentage of protein, fat, and carbohydrate is not significantly altered by cooking. As the calculated values have been rounded to whole numbers, and are affected by various other factors, the percentages given here may not in every case total 100%.

scientists clearly proved that strenuous activity involves no increased use of protein. Unfortunately, the prevailing nutritional viewpoint is that athletes need high-fat, high protein foods for strength and endurance.

Recently, a practice known as "carbohydrate loading" has become popular as a way of increasing the stamina of long-distance runners and other endurance athletes. Carbohydrate loading originated in 1967 when Dr. Per-Olof Astrand, an exercise physiologist from Stockholm, tested nine Swedish athletes for endurance on a stationary bicycle. After three days on a diet high in grains and vegetables, the athletes were, on the average, able to pedal three times longer than they did after three days on a diet high in meat and animal fats. In measuring the level of glycogen (fuel held in reserve) in the athletes' thigh muscles, Astrand found 3.51 grams per 100 grams of muscle after the vegetarian diet, compared with 1.75 grams after the three days on the high-fat, high-protein diet. From Dr. Astrand's experiment, and others like it, the concept of carbohydrate loading emerged.

Carbohydrate loading takes a week to complete. Seven days before an athletic event, the athlete will train until totally exhausted to deplete muscle and liver glycogen. For the next three days he or she will eat as many high-protein or high-fat foods (such as red meat, eggs, poultry, and milk) as possible, with a minimum of carbohydrates. For the three days immediately preceding competition, the athlete's diet consists of high-carbohydrate, low-fat, low-protein foods such as pasta, bread, grains, sweets, and so on, in small meals throughout the day. During this carbohydrate loading phase, the muscles and liver store a relative overload of glycogen, which is needed for stamina and endurance on the day of the competition.

Though the practice of carbohydrate loading has met with some success, it is not without its dangers. The high-protein, high-fat phase of the diet creates ketones—toxic substances which can lead to dehydration and kidney damage. In addition, the carbohydrate loading phase may bring large amounts of fat into the blood. Should the athlete have an existing heart condition, the rise in blood fats could cause a heart attack.

The best way to improve athletic performance, especially endurance, is to adopt the macrobiotic diet. Since it is naturally high in complex carbohydrates, the muscles will store the optimal amount of glycogen, without shocking the system.

A DIET FOR ENDURANCE

Vegetarian animals such as horses, giraffes, and antelope have greater endurance than carnivores such as the members of the cat family, who are known for their long, lazy naps. This relationship of diet to endurance appears to hold true for humans as well.

The Tarahumara Indians, who live in the Sierra Madre mountains of northwestern Mexico, are an example of almost completely vegetarian super-athletes. Their diet consists almost entirely of beans, corn, squash, pumpkins, root vegetables, wild plants, and fruits, with only occasional animal food (about one percent of their diet). Yet they may be the world's greatest endurance athletes.

Their bodies are strong and lean, and they are great runners. In their local sport, a kind of soccer game played with an oak ball the size of a baseball, the players run up to two hundred miles before the game ends. During the night, other runners light the path with torches. The runners stop only every dozen miles or so for food and water. William E. Connor, who studied the Tarahumaras extensively, found them to be remarkably healthy. He reported his findings in the *American Journal of Clinical Nutrition* in 1979 and 1982.

Closer to home, a number of successful athletes and super-athletes follow a diet high in complex carbohydrates and low in fat and protein, similar to the macrobiotic diet.

World class marathon runner Rob de Castella, winner of the 1982 Commonwealth Games in Brisbane, Australia, and the 1983 Fukuoka marathon in Japan; Martina Navratilova, the world's top-seeded women's tennis player; David Scott, the greatest triathlete in the world (competing in a ten-hour swimming, bicycling, and running competition); Scott Molina and Scott Tinley, two of Scott's closest competitors in the triathlon; and Jack Stevens, current world record holder for the 400, 800, and 1600 meter races in the 65-69 age group, are just a few of the athletes mentioned in Nathan Pritikin's 1984 book *The Pritikin Promise.* Sports enthusiasts can undoubtedly think of many others.

PROTEIN SOURCES AND WORLD HUNGER

Beyond the question of individual dietary needs, there is the larger problem of food shortage and world hunger. The heavy drain on the world's energy and natural resources points to the need for a wide-scale re-evaluation of our attitudes toward, and dependence upon, animal proteins as dietary staples. In modern practice, whole foods are often concentrated into refined and relatively less nutritious products. An average fast food meal is an example. It takes nearly ten pounds of grain to produce the beef from which a hamburger is made; thirty ears of corn to get the oil for French fries; four pounds of soybeans and a half-quart of milk to make a shake; more than one pound of beets to produce enough sugar to sweeten a dessert; a host of additives to improve the flavor, texture, and shelf life of fast foods; and two grams of salt to flavor them. In addition, many refined foods which are high in saturated fats and calories are low in naturally occurring vitamins and minerals.

In the United States, nearly two thousand pounds of grain are consumed per person every year (directly and through food for livestock). People in the rest of the world average about four hundred pounds of grain per year. Tufts University president Dr. Jean Mayer is outspoken when it comes to our dependence on meat as food. Dr. Mayer estimates that reducing meat consumption by just 10 percent annually would release enough grain to feed sixty million people.

Frances Moore Lappé, the author of *Diet For A Small Planet*, points out that North Americans, who make up about 7 percent of the world's population, consume over 30 percent of the world's animal foods. She contends that producing meat to supply humans with protein is grossly inefficient, and shows how vast acreage of land presently used to raise livestock could feed up to twenty times more people if planted with food crops instead.

Vegetarian Baseball Team

A Japanese baseball team climbed from the cellar to first place by switching to a macrobiotic diet.

Beginning in October 1981, when he took over as manager of the Seibu Lions, Tatsuro Hirooka prescribed a dietary change for his players, who had finished in last place the previous season. Hirooka limited their meat intake and banned polished rice and sugar altogether. Instead, he said, his players would eat unpolished rice, tofu, fish and soybean milk. The following spring, he ordered them onto a vegetable and soy diet.

Hirooka told his men that meats and other "animal foods" increase an athlete's susceptibility to injuries. Natural foods, on the other hand, protect the body from sprains and dislocations and keep the mind clear.

The Lions took a lot of ribbing during the 1982 season. The manager of the Nippon-Ham Fighters—a team sponsored by a major meat company—called the Lions "the goat team" and sneered, "They are only eating weeds." But the Lions edged out the Ham Fighters for the Pacific League championship in what sportswriters called the "Vegetable vs. Meat War," then went on to beat the Chunichi Dragons in the Japan Series. Seibu again won the Pacific League championship and the Japan Series in 1983. Food for thought, isn't it?■

"Significa" from *Parade Magazine*, April 1984, by Irving Wallace, David Wallechinsky, Amy Wallace. Reprinted by permission.

Fats and the
Macrobiotic Diet

The human body stores any extra energy that is supplied by the diet as fat. As the modern diet is too high in both fat and total calories, it tends to foster excessive weight gain. Two of every three adults in the United States are significantly overweight. More than fifty million people in this country are either on a diet or are contemplating one. This chapter will compare the sources of fats in the modern diet with those in the macrobiotic diet. Several areas in which dietary fat consumption is of particular interest—overweight, heart disease, and infant nutrition—will be discussed.

For many people the struggle to maintain normal weight begins slowly. Between the ages of twenty-five and forty they accumulate an extra fourteen pounds of fat. In many cases, this gain of one pound per year will occur even if only forty extra calories (above the daily average of two thousand) are consumed. The extra calories can be visualized as just one extra teaspoon of sugar per day. Twenty minutes of slow walking or ten minutes of brisk walking every day would help to neutralize these extra calories. A change of diet could eliminate them altogether. The macrobiotic diet includes more whole grains, vegetables, and beans than the typical modern diet does, and fewer sources of fat.

Most physicians agree that being overweight poses significant risks to health. Not because of any psychological drain it may have on the overweight individual, but strictly because being too heavy is a menace to physical health. According to the panel of scientists who reported to the Senate Select Committee on Nutrition and Human Needs a few years ago, obesity increases the risk of developing heart disease and hypertension (high blood pressure), gall bladder disease, and certain forms of cancer. It also aggravates arthritis, damages the liver, increases the risk of hernia, and causes difficulty in pregnancy and childbirth.

THE MACROBIOTIC DIET AND WEIGHT LOSS

Although many complex explanations are frequently offered for why and how individuals become overweight in the first place, it is really quite simple: they eat too much of the wrong kinds of foods and they don't exercise enough. The modern diet is about 42 percent fat (mostly saturated animal fat), which has more than twice the calories of protein or complex carbohydrates. Food processing has also condensed many of the foods commonly eaten. Since their bulk (natural food fiber) is removed, it is easier to fit more food—and calories—into the stomach in less time.

On the macrobiotic diet, up to 10 percent of an average meal is bulk, compared with about 2 percent or less in the diet eaten by most people today. The added bulk gives a satisfied feeling of being full, without adding calories to the diet. It also helps the body to more quickly and efficiently eliminate the food it does not use.

Unlike the foods that comprise the popular high-protein weight loss diets, which tend to drain energy and stimulate cravings for sweets, the complex carbohydrates in the macrobiotic diet reduce cravings for sweets and other fattening foods, and provide plenty of energy as well.

Losing weight and then maintaining the desired weight is not difficult on the macrobiotic diet. As a group, people who shun foods high in saturated fats (such as red meats, dairy products, and poultry), and simple sugars, are trim—and tend to stay that way. Depending on how much you weigh now and the extent to which you adhere to macrobiotic principles, your weight should normalize in a matter of days, weeks, or months. As in William Dufty's case, fifty or more pounds lost over a period of months is not uncommon.

On the macrobiotic diet, as long as you eat until satisfied, two or three times per day, you will meet your bodily nutritional needs. You can generally expect to lose about one to three pounds a week. Of course, if you also begin even a moderate exercise program (see Chapter 10) your results will be enhanced. As an added bonus your blood fat and cholesterol levels, and your blood pressure, will normalize as well.

THE FATS WITHIN

The excessive dietary intake of cholesterol and fats creates significant health risks. As you probably know, cholesterol, a substance akin to fats, has been implicated in coronary disease. In the past few years, many people have cut down on the amount of saturated animal fats they consume, and reduced their cholesterol intake. However, the consumption of highly refined vegetable oils and hydrogenated vegetable fats (oils saturated with hydrogen) such as margarine and shortening, has increased. And while these polyunsaturated vegetable fats are considered more healthful by many experts, the total fat content of the average diet is still too high, regardless of its food sources.

Even unrefined vegetable oils, if consumed in excess, can create blood too rich in fat and cholesterol. Most often the result is artery damage or atherosclerosis, a degenerative disease characterized by the development of plaques and fibrous tissue lining (and in most cases blocking) the artery walls. Heart disease, as this condition is commonly referred to, is the number one killer in America.

THE MACROBIOTIC SOLUTION TO HEART DISEASE

Separate studies by Kass and Sacks (1974, 1982), Bergin and Brown (1982), *The East West Journal* (1980), and Knuiman and West (1982) have shown the macrobiotic diet to be effective in reducing elevated blood fat and cholesterol levels to healthy levels. It had a similar effect on high blood pressure, returning it to normal. In a 1981 study conducted by Sacks et al., twenty-one healthy "macrobiotic eaters" were given beef for thirty days to determine the effect of meat and saturated animal fat on normal, healthy blood fat and cholesterol levels. In two weeks the subjects' blood cholesterol rose on the average from 140 mg/dl (milligrams per deciliter) before the test to 166 mg/dl after. Blood pressure also increased significantly.

Shortly after the individuals returned to the macrobiotic diet, their cholesterol and blood pressure returned to their previous levels. Clearly the macrobiotic diet is a promising solution to heart disease.

Of course, some fat is necessary and even healthful. The oils found naturally occurring in whole foods, and those oils which are extracted from whole foods without further refining, are the most healthful types. In moderate quantities, they help to protect the nerves from degeneration and lubricate the blood and the passage-ways it flows through. They also serve as emergency fuel reserves, keeping the body warmer in cold weather, and converting to energy when stores of glycogen are low. A little oil used in making bread or to sauté vegetables will improve the food's flavor and digestibility as well.

Of the polyunsaturated fats, unrefined corn and sesame oils are the most stable oils for use in cooking and baking. They are follow-ed by safflower, olive, and the other oils we will discuss in Chapter 8. Stability is the capacity of an oil to retain its freshness on the store shelf or in your cupboard. The naturally occurring Vitamin E found in unrefined oils contributes to their stability, serving as a preserva-tive against rancidity.

About 10 to 15 percent of the calories in the macrobiotic diet come from fats. This reflects an ideal balance.

FATS IN DAIRY PRODUCTS

The quality of milk and dairy food today is very different from that consumed by traditional peoples. Pasteurization, homogenization, and the addition of synthetic Vitamin D chemically alter milk prod-ucts. In addition, traditional peoples such as the Abkhasians, who use some dairy products, almost always ferment them. Cultured products such as yogurt and kefir are superior to other dairy prod-ucts because they are more easily broken down in the digestive pro-cess. However, even cultured dairy products are not usually recom-mended for regular consumption on the macrobiotic diet, because they contain excessive amounts of saturated fats and cholesterol.

Recent research published in *Diet, Nutrition, and Cancer*, a Nation-al Academy of Sciences report, has linked the fats in dairy products to an increase in the presence of cysts and tumors of the breast, uterus, and ovaries in American women. Japanese women, who rarely consume dairy foods, and who eat fewer saturated fats, have a lower incidence of these problems.

In addition, many people find that dairy foods cause the body to produce excess mucus, which often appears as postnasal drip, symptoms of allergies, breathing difficulties, and blockage or irritation of the sinuses. The minimal use or complete avoidance of dairy foods has, in many cases, caused a reversal of these and other related problems.

Allergies to Grains

The fats and proteins in dairy products may be responsible for some food allergies. Through the years I have counseled many people who, for one reason or another, were allergic to whole grains. In my opinion, people who are allergic either to the gluten or to other components of wheat, oats, corn, noodles, cereals, or flour products have probably been consuming too many dairy products as well as too much sugar since birth. How much is too much? Almost any amount, if there is an allergy to whole grains. Most likely the problem begins in infancy.

Babies fed cow's milk or formula miss out on their mother's colostrum, the milk secreted in the first few days after an infant's birth. Colostrum is needed to create strong immunity and healthy intestinal flora (bacteria) before the baby is ready to digest solid foods. Formula-fed babies are much more prone to disease in childhood, and to food allergies later on—especially if they continue to consume excessive amounts of dairy foods and sugar.

Years of eating these foods cause a change in the cells of the stomach and intestines, including the villi (small tentacle-like structures which are responsible for assimilating food). The entire body may adapt to the larger protein molecules found in cow's milk and the excesses of calcium and other nutrients it supplies. At the same time it may develop adverse reactions to normally wholesome foods, and we call these reactions allergies.

If you are presently allergic to glutenous grains, especially wheat, oats, or corn, try using brown rice or millet, which are lower in gluten, as substitutes. Also increase the amount of vegetables you eat, and eat more beans and bean products as well. Gradually reduce the amount of dairy products and sugary foods in the diet until you are able to avoid them completely. In a few weeks, try eating a small amount of the glutenous whole grains. In time, it may become possible for you to digest and assimilate whole grains without any adverse reactions.

The Best Sources of Dietary Calcium

Many people who were raised on cow's milk have come to depend upon it as a source of dietary calcium. However, as you can see from Table 4.1, which lists various sources of calcium in the macrobiotic diet, many foods besides milk are rich sources of this vital mineral. And since these foods are all of vegetable origin, they offer higher-quality nutrition for adults—they contain less saturated fat and cholesterol.

Calcium regulates heartbeat, blood clotting, and overall mineral balance. It also builds healthy teeth and bones. Osteoporosis, a progressive weakening of the bones, frequently leads to fractures and death. American women over thirty-five years of age are particularly susceptible to this condition. While many complex explanations have been offered as to the cause of osteoporosis, it is most likely due to high protein intake together with the excessive consumption of simple sugars. This modern diet causes calcium and other minerals stored in the bones to be reabsorbed into the bloodstream. By supplying an optimum amount of protein and a variety of calcium-rich foods, the macrobiotic diet can help remedy this condition without side effects.

MACROBIOTIC INFANT NUTRITION

Milk has always served as a vital link between generations. Through the mother-infant breastfeeding relationship, the foundation was laid for the unfolding of intelligence and human consciousness. Even today the long dependency of the newborn upon its mother tightens the bond between them and ensures that the child grows strong and healthy.

Research compiled over the past twenty years has proved beyond a reasonable doubt that mother's milk is best for newborn babies. Formula-fed babies are more likely to develop digestive

Table 4.1 Calcium Sources

Calcium Source	Serving Size	Calcium (mg.) Per Serving	Calcium (mg.) Per 100 g.
Leafy Green Vegetables			
Broccoli, steamed	1 cup	136	103
Mustard greens, steamed	1 cup	193	140
Turnip greens, steamed	1 cup	267	184
Kale, steamed	1 cup	282	185
Collards, steamed	1 cup	357	188
Seeds, Nuts, and Beans			
Sunflower seeds	2½ ounces	45	120
Pinto beans, dried	4 ounces	67	135
Chick peas, dried	4 ounces	75	150
Tofu	3½ ounces	154	154
Almonds	2½ ounces	167	234
Dairy*			
Whole milk	1 cup	291	118
Cheddar cheese	1 ounce	204	750
Sea Vegetables			
Dulse	2 tablespoons	—	296
Agar-agar	2 tablespoons	—	567
Irish moss	2 tablespoons	—	885
Kelp	2 tablespoons	—	1093

*Not generally recommended for use on the macrobiotic diet.

Sources: United States Department of Agriculture and Japan Nutritionist Association.

Note: A dash signifies that data is not available.

problems and diarrhea. They also have a lowered immunity to illness and infection, and less of a chance of surviving the first years of life alive and well.

Mother's milk is the best way to protect infants from viruses and microbes. It gives them a solid immunity against infection. According to Arthur Guyton, M.D., a noted medical physiologist and the author of the *Textbook of Medical Physiology*, mother's milk contains specific antibodies that combat the growth of undesirable bacteria and viruses. Leonard J. Mata, in *Uniqueness of Human Milk*, says that mother's milk protects babies against rickettsia (which can cause fever and typhus), polio, influenza virus, salmonella, microbes that can cause intestinal infection, staph, strep, and other infections.

In addition, a child's intelligence may also be limited by the use of cow's milk. Studies reported in an article by W.B. Whitestone, entitled *Biological Specificity Of Milk*, and published by La Leche League in 1976, have shown that breast-fed children develop better reading and spelling skills than their counterparts who are fed cow's milk. It is not so difficult to understand why this could be so.

All creatures are born at different stages of biological development. For example, many species of fish can swim and eat immediately after they are born. Horses and cows are able to stand just hours after birth. Human babies can do little more than suck, and are totally dependent on their mothers for a much longer time than most other animals.

Using brain development as a guide, we can compare the different animals and their nutritional needs in infancy. At birth, the human brain is about 23 percent developed, compared with 40 percent in the chimpanzee and gorilla. A calf's brain is nearly 100 percent developed by the time the calf first sees the light of day. The various animals continue to show different rates of brain development after birth as well. Within the first year of life, the chimp's brain is three-quarters developed, but it takes three years for the human baby to reach the same developmental stage.

Not needing much brain food, but rather food for bone and muscle building, the calf may gain seventy-five pounds in the first six weeks. Cow's milk is three times richer in protein and contains four times more calcium than human milk. Human infants, on the other hand, grow less than a pound a week during the first six weeks. An infant's need for protein and calcium is much less than that of a baby calf. However, his or her requirement for carbohydrates, which nourish nerve and brain cells, is much greater than the calf's—and human mother's milk contains nearly twice as much carbohydrates as cow's milk.

While the practice of giving newborn babies cow's milk has been abandoned in recent years, some mothers still introduce cow's milk when their babies are a few months old. This may lead to long-term health problems, as cow's milk is too rich in protein, calcium, and other minerals. It was created this way to support the growth and development of a three-hundred pound calf.

Children fed cow's milk may become bigger in size more quickly, but their internal organs become somewhat lazy, loose, and enlarged. As it is composed of larger molecules than mother's milk, cow's milk tends to overnourish the body and undernourish the brain and nervous system. Breast-fed babies are generally brighter, more sensitive and more alert than those fed cow's milk.

In most parts of the world, little milk is drunk by children over two years of age. Only by a lifetime of constant milk-drinking have some Europeans and Americans developed a seeming tolerance for dairy foods. Part of the reason that many people continue to use milk, butter, cheese, yogurt, and ice cream is habit, and part is emotional need. Just as babies are reluctant to give up breastfeeding and the taste and texture of milk, adults tend to develop an emotional attachment to its substitutes. The addiction goes beyond the emotions, however; as we have seen, the body is changed physically by years of dairy use.

Macrobiotic infant care suggests that the mother decrease the amount of breastfeeding when the child reaches about six months of age, while introducing soft foods such as creamy cooked brown rice cereal, millet, mashed noodles, oatmeal, soft cooked and mashed beans, vegetables, sea vegetables, and fruit. During the next year, the child is gradually weaned to soft foods. Harder foods can be introduced at around twenty to twenty-four months. Fruits and whole grain cookies replace candies and sugared foods in the macrobiotic diet, and children can enjoy them with tea or amasake (a fermented drink made from sweet brown rice), instead of milk. Soymilk or nut/seed milk, beans and bean products, and whole grain drinks such as amasake will make good replacements for dairy products during the transition to a more macrobiotic diet.

5

Fiber, Fermented Foods, and Digestion

The increased consumption of refined foods, sugar, and red meats, has led to a drastic increase in problems of the lower digestive tract. The average American diet is extremely low in fiber, and also has an adverse effect upon the beneficial microbes present in the colon (large intestine). To prevent eliminative problems, including colon cancer, macrobiotics suggests the use of whole foods such as whole grains, beans, and vegetables, which are rich in fiber, and fermented foods such as miso, tempeh, tamari, umeboshi, sauerkraut, and pickles.

Speaking before a group of doctors, British M.D. Dennis Burkitt, an authority on dietary fiber, explained our failing health in simple terms. Americans, he noted, have small stools and big hospitals. That is, due to a fiber-deficient diet, Americans suffer from a number of problems of the digestive tract, ranging from tooth decay to constipation and colon-rectal cancer (which is the third leading cause of death in the United States).

Fiber is perhaps the least understood portion of the food we eat. For years it was believed to be a useless non-nutrient that should be removed from foods to make them more digestible and palatable. In recent years, however, doctors and scientists such as Dennis Burkitt have extensively studied the role of fiber in nutrition. Their conclusion is that, on the average, we cannot live very healthy or long lives without it.

FIBER AND FIBER DEFICIENCY

Fiber is the skeleton of the plant—the part that provides structural support. Every plant cell is surrounded by a fibrous wall. Fiber also forms part of the seeds, leaves, and stems. It is not a single substance, but is composed of three different groups of substances: pentoses, which are complex carbohydrates; cellulose, which is also a complex carbohydrate; and lignin, a woody component.

Whereas fats, proteins, and non-fibrous carbohydrates are almost entirely absorbed in the small intestine, fiber moves through the colon, or large intestine, virtually unchanged. As it is not digested in the usual sense, Westerners have been refining foods to remove their fiber for over a hundred years.

In reality, fiber affects the function of the entire alimentary tract, exerting its greatest influence in the colon. Fiber adds bulk to the feces, facilitating their transit through the intestines. It also inhibits the formation of toxins and the growth of certain harmful bacteria in the colon. By diluting the concentration of toxins, fiber also prevents the colon wall from being harmed.

Oriental peoples and those living in developing nations do not suffer from bowel disorders to the same extent that Americans do because their diet is less refined and includes more vegetables and fiber-rich foods. The incidence of colon cancer in the United States is 900 percent higher than in Nigeria and 1300 percent greater than in Uganda, two countries in which the diet is traditionally high in fiber. Yet after two generations of living in the U.S., American blacks contract colon cancer at the same rate as American whites. Second generation Japanese-Americans living in Hawaii, having left their traditional high-fiber diet, also contract colon cancer at the same rate as the rest of the American public.

MACROBIOTICS AND FIBER

There is much evidence suggesting that switching to a high-fiber diet can prevent eliminative disorders such as constipation, hemorrhoids, diverticular disease, colitis, and bowel cancer. Fiber-rich foods such as whole grains may also prevent tooth decay, diabetes, obesity, heart disease, high blood cholesterol levels, varicose veins, and liver and gall bladder problems.

The macrobiotic diet is high in fiber, and is the best way to promote a number of positive changes in the body. When someone eats macrobiotically, the muscles of the colon are strengthened. In addition, the stools become larger, less-hard packed, and easier to pass. They contain at least three times more fiber than the average person's. Also, the intestinal flora (bacteria in the intestine) becomes more healthy and more acidic, preventing gas and putrefaction. Not only is dietary change more effective than laxatives in correcting problems of the bowel, it is the only really safe and long-lasting solution there is.

FIBER CONTENT OF FOODS

Fiber is more abundant on the outside surfaces of whole grains, seeds, beans, vegetables, and fruits, than on the inside. The bran of whole grains, and the skins of beans, vegetables, and fruits contain large amounts of fiber. This is one important reason why the macrobiotic diet recommends using whole rather than polished grains, and unpeeled fruits and vegetables (whenever possible).

Many people, recognizing the importance of fiber, use bran, which is 44 percent fiber, as a dietary supplement. However, added bran is not recommended for regular consumption as it may irritate the colon wall, and block the absorption of nutrients provided by other foods. Whole grains, beans, seeds, nuts, and unpeeled vegetables and fruits have an ideal balance of fiber and other nutrients. By eating plenty of these foods you will get three or four times the fiber supplied by the average modern diet. Table 5.1 compares the fiber content of various foods. Animal products have been omitted as most of them contain little or no fiber.

Table 5.1   Fiber Content of Foods

Item	Percent Fiber	Item	Percent Fiber
Bran	44.0	Greens (average)	3.8
Almonds	15.0	Carrots	3.1
Soybeans	14.3	Broccoli	3.0
Green peas	12.0	Brussels sprouts	2.9
Whole wheat	9.6	Apples	2.0
Whole meal bread	8.5	White flour	2.0
Peanuts	8.1	White potato	2.0
Pinto beans	7.0	White rice	0.8
Beans, other	7.0	Grapefruit	0.6
Raisins	6.8	Orange juice	0.5
Brown rice	5.5	Sugar	0.0
Lentils	3.8		

FERMENTED FOODS

Equally as important as keeping the muscles and walls of the colon in good shape with a steady supply of dietary fiber is keeping the flora inside it healthy. Though little is known about the fifty trillion microbes inside our intestines, what we do know could prevent much suffering and save some lives.

When we digest our food, it not only feeds us, but also feeds the bacteria in the intestines. Whole grains, vegetables, and especially fermented foods such as sauerkraut, pickles, umeboshi plums, miso, tamari, sourdough breads, amasake, and tempeh, produce lactic acid in the colon. This acid gently tones the colon and corrects the balance between beneficial digestive bacteria and those potentially harmful but active bacteria that cannot develop so effectively in an acid medium.

The protective action of lactic-acid-producing foods was pointed out in a study of Japanese-Americans by J. Clark, published in the *Western Journal of Medicine* (1974). Clark found that Americans of Japanese descent still living on their traditional Japanese diet, including about two tablespoons of miso per day, along with other traditional fermented foods, had a significantly different and simpler (less diverse) population of microbes in their intestines, compared to average Americans.

W. Morre and L. Holderman, writing in *Cancer Research* (1975), also reported a lower incidence of certain illnesses, especially bowel cancer, in populations where the bacterial flora is simpler than ours. The rural Africans and the rural Japanese are good examples of people with a more simple diet who have few eliminative problems. A simple grain-based diet of mostly unrefined foods, combined with the regular use of lactic-acid-producing fermented foods, and minimal consumption of meat and dairy products, is the key to their relative freedom from intestinal disorders, including colon cancer.

Light and salty tasting miso soup, made with miso paste and vegetables, is a popular broth that can be eaten at least once a day on the macrobiotic diet. Tempeh, another fermented food commonly eaten on the macrobiotic diet, is made from soybeans. Pickled cucumbers, which you can easily make yourself at home, are another favorite, as is old-fashioned sauerkraut made with cabbage and sea salt. We will have more to say about the uses and preparation of these and other fermented foods later.

Dirk Benedict's Toughest Battle

William Dufty, author of Sugar Blues, *which blames sugar for all kinds of health problems, introduced Benedict to Boston-based macrobiotics expert Michio Kushi. Benedict says Kushi's teachings saved his life.*

In a recent medical exam Benedict received a clean bill of health from Dr. Keith Block of Evanston, Ill., who says, "In my opinion, his recovery is remarkable. Considering his age, it's very unlikely the tumor was benign." Benedict decided to talk with Lois Armstrong about the several cross-country journeys and the diet that changed his life.

I used to eat like a horse. I'd have venison steak, eggs and pancakes for breakfast, meat loaf for lunch and a big steak, potatoes, salad and apple pie or a piece of cake for dinner. I ate what Hemingway wrote about. In college I was a 200-pound linebacker, but I had very bad arthritis in my knees, hips and hands, and headaches, hair loss and skin problems. Then in 1971, while I was in Sweden doing a movie, I quit eating meat and chicken, and within 10 days the pains in my knees stopped. In 1972 I began building my entire diet around grains, and by the end of 1974, I had stopped eating dairy foods.

When I gave up meat, I was floundering. I was reading books on diet and Eastern philosophy and medicine, pursuing alternative ways of caring for yourself but for strictly physical reasons. Then Gloria and Bill introduced me to the Oriental philosophy behind an alternate way of eating—macrobiotics. Yin and yang. The balance of opposing yet complementary forces. They saved me years of searching.

In May of 1975 I was told I had prostate trouble. I'd had pain and was passing blood. But I'd already changed my way of eating and I was thinking in much healthier terms.

I was so pleased, having thick hair and no arthritis. My whole body had changed. I just didn't believe this could happen.

One doctor told me I had a tumor of the prostate, and then I went to another doctor in New York who said, "Yes. Definitely." He wanted to slap me right into the hospital. Bill Dufty had gone with me to the doctor. The way Bill figured it: "If they decide you have a problem, you're never going to get out of there. They'll lock you up and go to work." Bill was right. After the doctor gave me the bad news, some people came in with forms to fill out to check me into the hospital. I backed out of the office and down the hallway with doctors yelling after me. It was a scene right out of *General Hospital.*

Then I went to see Michio Kushi in Boston. I had met him three years before through Miss Swanson. He confirmed that I had a prostate tumor and said it was very important for me "to have good behavior" for the next four months by sticking with the diet. No cheating. I was not scared because I had been studying macrobiotics, and I believed completely in the principles behind it. Actually, I was excited by the adventure of it. Growing up in Montana, I learned: If the tractor breaks down, fix it. So I always have had that in my nature. It was dangerous, but I wanted to figure it out on my own.

I didn't know what I was in store for. I didn't know how painful the journey was going to be, how difficult. I know people who've tried macrobiotic treatment for awhile, and then just gone back to their cheesecakes. Everybody wants to be cured, but they want it to be easy, and they want it to be fast.

When I learned I had a tumor—I refused to be tested for malignancy—I weighed 180 pounds. When I came out of the mountains of New Hampshire six weeks later, I weighed 155. I went to stay in a friend's cabin because I didn't want any distractions, any temptations, anybody calling up to say, "Let's go have a bagel." Well, all hell broke loose. Some days I felt on top of the world, and other days I couldn't get out of bed. Sometimes I couldn't walk up the stairs, and sometimes I'd ride, run and chop wood for 24 hours.

I wore a swimsuit all the time. There was no one around and no full-length mirrors—so I was shocked when I put on a pair of pants and they fell right off. I continued to lose weight, down to 135 pounds, at which point there were people who wanted to get me into a hospital. I looked like exactly what I was, someone who was seriously ill.

I never did go into a hospital. Instead, I packed up my duffel bag and became a vagabond, traveling to Montana, Maine, California, New York City, Wisconsin, hitchhiking across the country once and driving across twice. I wrote short stories, a couple of screen treatments and a proposal for a TV series. Food was a problem, though. The only thing I could find to eat in restaurants was oatmeal. I'd ask for one bowl, then another, and finally I'd ask for it in a salad bowl. The rest of the time, I relied on a little cast-iron pot, cooking grains and vegetables in the open field.

I shouldn't have traveled. I should have stayed in one place and taken care of myself. My body was starving to death. I was not eating anything my body was used to. Because of the cancer fear, I was not cheating. Before that, I would have a little cheese, a little fish, bread, salad, but now all that was gone. I was eating only grains, so my body was living off my fat, and then my body was eating my muscles. It was taking the protein out of my muscles; in effect, I was consuming myself. I used to dream about hamburgers and steaks pleading with me to eat them, like a Walt Disney nightmare.

At one point, I was driving from L.A. to the East Coast, and I swung up to Montana to see my family. I probably shouldn't have done that. I had never told them of my condition. It doesn't matter now, but I couldn't say it then. When my mother, who works in a hospital, saw how thin I was, she pleaded with me to see a doctor. I left her and my sister sobbing in the backyard and went down the road to New York.

I began to feel I was getting better when the weight started coming back after about a year on the diet. I weighed 135 until the end of 1975, and then I went up to 148 halfway through 1976. I even stuck to the diet while I was doing *Battlestar Galactica* in 1978, but I was actually a little pudgy by then. It was at that point that I felt I was beginning to recover. About two months ago, I got my passing grade from Dr. Block after extensive blood tests. I don't have the tumor anymore.

With macrobiotics, you begin to sense what *you* want. Most mornings now I have Japanese miso soup—which is made with soybean paste, chunks of tofu, seaweed and scallions—and a big bowl of oatmeal. I take my own lunch to the studio—some kind of steamed vegetable. I also eat a lot of pasta and winter squashes. From the world of vegetables, there's almost nothing I don't eat. About 60 percent of my diet is grain, about 25 percent beans and another 15 percent side dishes like nuts, seeds, fruit and fish. That's about as wide as I go.

The thing this diet does give you is stamina and endurance. What it does not give you is tremendous bulk strength. It wouldn't be too good for Mr. T. Some weightlifter friends of mine recently helped me move furniture. In the beginning they were stronger, but after two hours, I was still strong and they were pooped.

And my love life has changed. I appreciate a different kind of woman. I think the whole *Playboy* thing is the result of a meat-eating mentality. It's a gratification that is purely physical. It doesn't incorporate the emotional, the mental, the spiritual aspects of the female. But it doesn't have to be like that. I have a girlfriend now, Toni Hudson—she's in *Cross Creek* and next she's going to do a film in Texas with Sally Field—and she cooks and makes my lunch. Toni's a very secure individual in her female identity. She appreciates the maleness in me and finds it exciting rather than threatening. She eats this food too, and she's gone from thin to thinner. My weight now has stabilized at 155 to 160 pounds. At 5'11", I weigh what I weighed as a teenager.

Macrobiotics is not to be taken lightly. It's not like going to see Richard Simmons twice a week and bouncing around and eating your salad. If you want to try macrobiotics, get some literature on the subject and read it. If it makes sense, incorporate it to some extent. Maybe three times a week, instead of having meat, eat brown rice. The whole point of macrobiotics is to get control of your life, and then deal with it yourself. Life belongs to those who are willing to accept the responsibility for having it. ■

Reported by Lois Armstrong, *People Weekly,* October 10, 1983, Time Inc. Reprinted by permission.

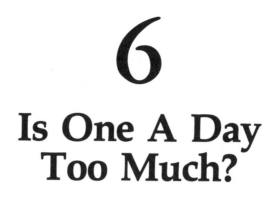

6

Is One A Day Too Much?

Among nutritional and scientific circles there are two opposing sides to the question of whether vitamin and mineral supplements are necessary. There are those who say it is foolish to use supplements; that the average diet supplies all the micro-nutrients (vitamins, minerals, and trace elements) that we need. And there are those who tell us it's better to use supplements because we have nutritional deficiencies due to poor diet and environmental stresses.

The American public has the highest micro-nutrient intake in the world, due to the widespread use of vitamin and mineral supplements. A recent survey conducted by the Food and Drug Administration (FDA) indicated that over 60 million Americans believe that vitamin supplements are absolutely necessary for good health. In addition, the study reported that 20 million Americans believe that vitamin deficiency can lead to almost all diseases, including cancer.

Yet, in 1980 the National Academy of Sciences Committee on Dietary Allowances (the committee which established Recommended Daily Allowances, or RDAs) found no scientific evidence for nutritional benefits derived from vitamins, minerals, or trace elements in dosages greater than those supplied by a balanced diet.

One of the reasons that vitamin supplements are so popular is the massive advertising and promotion they receive (mostly sponsored by large pharmaceutical companies). Another reason is that there is some truth to the advertiser's claims. The human body does need vitamins and cannot do without them.

Vitamins are essential nutrients, not for energy purposes, but for their ability to regulate chemical reactions in the body. They help to make the energy present in food available for use. Without any vitamins we would starve. Without enough of the right kinds, our ability to process and use the nutrients in our diet is reduced, and a variety of deficiency symptoms, including malnutrition, may arise. Many people inadvertently destroy many vitamins that they consume in food. For example, washing with harsh soap strips away the Vitamin C that is part of the acid mantle protecting the skin. In addition, sugar and alcohol can neutralize the vitamins B_1, B_6, and folic acid. Smoking interferes with the body's uptake of Vitamin C. Excess protein or liquid in the diet can wash a variety of other vitamins out of the body, while antibiotics, laxatives, antacids, aspirin, many prescription drugs, and stress destroy even more.

Most of the vitamin supplements on the market are synthesized from coal tar and other petroleum derivatives. And while the synthetic substances may be chemically identical or closely related to the natural vitamins, they may have only a fraction of the biological activity. Synthetic vitamins may substitute for some, but not all, of the functions of their natural counterparts. Synthetics may also have additional effects beyond those of vitamins found in foods. In fact, vitamin manufacturers warn us that large doses of supplemental vitamins A, B complex, C, D, and E can harm the body. In addition, the use of smaller amounts of these synthetic vitamin supplements may lead to a gradual buildup of vitamin toxicity. If you do choose to use supplemental vitamins and minerals, try to obtain natural supplements (from food sources) rather than synthetic ones.

VITAMINS IN WHOLE FOODS

The macrobiotic diet supplies all the essential vitamins in quantities equal to or greater than the RDAs, without supplements. The key foods in the macrobiotic diet—whole grains, fresh vegetables and leafy greens, seeds, beans, and fruits, are among the most vitamin-rich foods known.

Vitamin A, which aids normal growth and development, is supplied in abundance on the macrobiotic diet in the form of beta carotene or pro-vitamin A. Pro-vitamin A is non-toxic even in large doses and is easily converted into usable Vitamin A by the liver.

Yellow and orange vegetables and leafy greens are excellent sources of pro-vitamin A.

The Vitamin B complex is a group of vitamins that work together. The B complex helps the body to digest and use the energy in carbohydrates, and fosters resistance to infection. Among the best natural sources of the B complex vitamins are whole grains, which comprise 50 percent of the macrobiotic diet.

Vitamin B_{12}, which is needed by the body in minute amounts (a few thousandths of a milligram per day), helps prevent nerve and cell degeneration, and aids in the formation of red blood cells. Since it is not found in plant tissue, it is sometimes perceived as lacking in the macrobiotic diet. However, it is often found as a bacteria or mold on the skins of organically grown fruits and vegetables. In cultures where food is organically grown and minimally processed, and where no eggs, meat, or milk is consumed, Vitamin B_{12} deficiency is rare. In addition, two important groups of supplementary macrobiotic foods—seafoods (such as sea vegetables, shellfish, white-meat fish), and soyfoods (especially tempeh and miso)—do contain small but significant amounts of Vitamin B_{12}.

Vitamin C has come to be regarded by many people as a panacea capable of curing the common cold, heart disease, cancer, and a number of other ailments. There is, however, no real evidence that extra supplemental Vitamin C does any of these things. It does protect the nerves, glands, and connective tissues from oxidation, and aid in the absorption of iron. The macrobiotic diet supplies three to five times the RDA for Vitamin C, which is 50 milligrams per day. The best natural sources of Vitamin C are leafy greens, broccoli, fresh fruits, and vegetables.

Vitamin D is not really a vitamin, as it is synthesized in the body. It plays a role in the body's absorption of calcium, and it is important to the health of bones and teeth. This vitamin is not normally taken in sufficient quantities from food alone—it is formed as a result of sunlight's action on certain cholesterol-like substances on the skin. Children in particular need regular exposure to sunlight. Fifteen to thirty minutes of facial exposure per day is sufficient.

Vitamin E is believed to be an antioxidant—a substance that protects important molecules and structures in the cell from being damaged by oxygen. Even though Vitamin E deficiency has never been observed in adult humans, supplemental Vitamin E is second only to Vitamin C in popularity. Advertisers claim supplemental Vitamin E increases sexual endurance, prevents heart attacks, and promotes longevity. Again, there is no evidence to support these claims. The RDA for Vitamin E, 10 milligrams per day, can be satisfied by the consumption of one cup of leafy greens. Whole grains, unrefined vegetable oils, seeds, nuts, and vegetables also contain healthful amounts of natural Vitamin E.

A varied macrobiotic diet provides more than enough vitamins to maintain optimal health, without the danger of vitamin toxicity or buildup.

ESSENTIAL VITAMINS AND WHAT THEY DO

The following table is intended to help you select the foods in your diet wisely. It lists good food sources for the most important vitamins, outlines their functions in the body, and compares the current Recommended Daily Allowances (RDAs) with the amounts supplied by a typical day on the macrobiotic diet.

MINERALS

Almost as many people who use vitamin pills each day use supplemental minerals. Minerals are added to white bread, cereals, canned foods, and baby foods. They can also be found among the vitamins in many supplements. But as is the case with most supplemental vitamins, the minerals added to foods or found in pills do not come from food sources at all, but rather from mines and quarries (via laboratories).

Minerals occurring naturally in food are always combined by nature with specific amino acids, and sometimes with a vitamin too. The body easily recognizes minerals in this form, and knows how to use them efficiently. As food additives or dietary supplements, however, minerals tend to confuse the body more than they help it.

When the body does accept a mineral element, it must then balance it with its overall mineral needs. Taking too much of a particular mineral can set up a chain reaction which unbalances all the other mineral levels. This doesn't mean that taking an iron pill for a few days will cause illness. It probably won't make any difference.

Table 6.1   Essential Vitamins and What They Do

Vitamin	Food Sources	Function in Body	RDA (adult)*	Estimated Macrobiotic Diet Value†
A (carotene)	alfalfa sprouts apricots carrots dandelion greens leafy greens orange and yellow vegetables parsley peaches winter squash	Aids normal growth, reproduction, and development. Aids skin, teeth, mucous membranes, and eyesight. Maintains resistance to infection.	5000 I.U.	14,789 I.U.
B₁ (thiamine)	beans leafy greens nuts seeds vegetables whole grains	Aids assimilation of starches and sugars; builds appetite and energy. Aids digestion, the heart, and the liver.	1.2–2.0 mg.	3.07 I.U.
B₂ (riboflavin)	almonds kelp leafy greens mushrooms soyfoods vegetables whole grains	Improves resistance to disease. Aids normal growth and development. Improves skin and eyesight.	1.6–2.6 mg.	1.85 mg.
B₁₂	bean sprouts dulse kombu soyfoods	Prevents nerve cell degeneration. Aids formation of red blood cells.	3–5 mcg.	5 mcg.

Sources:

*RDAs: the figures used are adapted from the RDAs established for adult males by the U.S. Food and Drug Administration in 1980.

†Estimated nutritional content of the Macrobiotic Diet (for one person, for one day) is based on *USDA Composition of Foods Handbook No. 8.*

Abbreviations used in the above table:
I.U.   — *International Units*
mg.   — *milligrams*
mcg. — *micrograms*

Note: A dash signifies that no RDA has been established.

Table 6.1—*Continued*

Vitamin	Food Sources	Function in Body	RDA (adult)*	Estimated Macrobiotic Diet Value†
Niacin (a B vitamin)	kelp leafy greens mushrooms peanuts and beans nuts sesame seeds sunflower seeds whole grains	Aids mental health and nervous system. Helps maintain appetite and adrenal health.	12–20 mg.	20.30 mg.
C (ascorbic acid)	broccoli Brussels sprouts cauliflower collards fruits kale parsley sprouts watercress	Aids growth and development. Maintains tissues, joints, ligaments, teeth, and gums. Promotes healing and resistance to infection.	75–100 mg.	236 mg.
D	fish sunlight	Promotes normal formation of strong bones and teeth.	400 I.U.	400 I.U.
E	leafy greens nuts and seeds vegetable oils whole grains	Aids reproduction, the heart, and the utilization of fatty acids.	10–30 mg.	20–45 mg.
K	alfalfa sprouts leafy greens sea vegetables vegetables whole grains	Aids blood coagulation. Decreases risk of hemorrhage in pregnancy.	—	300–500 mcg.

But if iron or other supplemental minerals are used over a longer period of time, they may upset all of the major mineral balances that are important to health.

Taking an iron pill to treat anemia actually may make the problem worse. When an individual takes an iron pill, his or her sodium level goes up due to adrenal stimulation. The elevated sodium lowers the magnesium level. This also brings the calcium down, the potassium up, and the copper and zinc down—ultimately lowering iron even further.

In other words, no mineral works alone; they all work in harmony to balance one another. Extreme diets, supplemental minerals, and some pathological conditions can overwhelm the delicate mechanisms that maintain the minerals in proper proportion. Healthy people eating a balanced whole foods diet will be able to keep their minerals in the proper ratio to one another. In fact, no matter what your physical condition is, food is the safest and best place from which to get all your minerals.

THE ROLE OF MINERALS IN HEALTH

The balanced minerals found in whole foods are extremely important. They help keep the energy level high, the nerves tranquil, and the muscles, heart, hair, and blood healthy. They are also important in the formation of bones, teeth, and nails. Moreover, minerals play a role in almost all of the physiological functions. For example, not only do they serve in maintaining immunity from disease, but also in regulating blood pH (the relative acidity or alkalinity of the blood). Just as sea water can neutralize toxins streaming into it from the land, minerals in our blood can neutralize excesses of acid or alkaline ash, the residue left behind from the digestion and metabolizing of foods.

Under normal circumstances our blood should maintain a slight alkalinity, having a pH between 7.3 and 7.45 (on the pH scale, below 7.0 is acid and above 7.0 is alkaline). As a result of metabolism, acids are constantly being produced. These must be neutralized by the alkaline elements in the blood, in order to prevent acidosis, ketosis shock, gout, and other problems. The more acid produced internally, and the more taken in from food, the lower the reserves of alkaline minerals like calcium will become. After years of a diet high in acid-forming foods such as red meat, sugar, poultry, eggs, tropical fruits, fats, and oils, the body becomes overly acidic. More calcium begins to leave the body than stays inside it, causing bones to weaken and teeth to decay.

Testing food for acidity or alkalinity is performed by burning the food and analyzing the ash that remains. If a food has an alkaline ash, it is alkaline, and if it has an acid ash, it is acid. The confusion surrounding the question of acid and alkaline foods regards the effect these foods have on the blood.

Some foods that test acid in ash—for example, whole grains, which have a mildly acidic ash—can actually have a slightly alkaline–forming effect on the blood. Alkaline ash foods such as tropical fruits, on the other hand, cause an acid reaction. Sugar, which is also alkaline ash, and some vegetables of tropical origin, including tomatoes, create acid in the blood as well.

Unlike the diet typical of many people today, the macrobiotic diet has a total pH value that is slightly alkaline-forming in the bloodstream. The result is a higher energy level, immunity from colds and flu, prevention of stomach upset, and stronger and more healthy bones and teeth.

Table 6.2 indicates good food sources of the essential minerals and details the functions of each in the body. It also compares the RDAs with the amounts supplied by a typical day on the macrobiotic diet.

Of all the foods we recommend you eat regularly, sea vegetables are the richest source of minerals. Millions of people all over the world still eat sea vegetables direct from the sea, and benefit both from the minerals they contain and the flavor they add to other foods. Table 6.3 lists the mineral content of the various sea vegetables recommended for regular consumption on the macrobiotic diet. The role of sea vegetables in the diet will be discussed more fully in the next chapter.

In this age of specialization, where the accumulated knowledge resulting from intense research is so great, it is easy to lose sight of the wholeness of life. This is not to say that knowledge of nutritional science is a waste of time. An understanding of nutritional needs can help us to better choose the whole foods we need and recognize when we need them. At the same time we must consciously look beyond fragments of truth to view the wholeness of life. Individuals born into a traditional way of life see no such separation. Their food selection is merely a part of their whole history, culture, and dietary tradition. And with their whole diet, these people preserve the wholeness of their health. In keeping with these traditions, the macrobiotic approach brings wholeness to our diet, and therefore to our health, and our lives.

Table 6.2   Essential Minerals and What They Do

Mineral	Food Sources	Function in Body	RDA (adult)*	Estimated Macrobiotic Diet Value†
Calcium	almonds daikon radish dandelion greens dulse kale kelp leafy greens nuts parsley sea vegetables sesame soyfoods watercress	Builds healthy bones and teeth. Helps blood clot. Regulates heartbeat and mineral balance.	800 mg.	859 mg.
Chlorine	celery green cabbage kale lettuce parsnips radishes sea vegetables vegetables	Aids digestion and elimination. Sustains normal heart activity.	trace	trace
Iodine	fish leafy greens sea vegetables vegetables (organically grown)	Stimulates thyroid gland, which regulates rate of digestion. Important for growth and development.	150 mcg.	150–300 mcg.

Sources:

*RDAs: the figures used are adapted from the RDAs established for adult males by the U.S. Food and Drug Administration in 1980.

†Estimated nutritional content of the Macrobiotic Diet (for one person, for one day) is based on *USDA Composition of Foods Handbook No. 8.*

Abbreviations used in the above table:
I.U. — *International Units*   mg. — *milligrams*   mcg. — *micrograms*

Note: A dash signifies that no RDA has been established.

Table 6.2—*Continued*

Mineral	Food Sources	Function in Body	RDA (adult)*	Estimated Macrobiotic Diet Value†
Iron	beans fruits (dried and fresh) kelp leafy greens nuts sea vegetables seeds tekka whole grains	Helps form hemoglobin and myoglobin. Aids oxygen transport to cells and prevents anemia.	10 mg.	39.3 mg.
Phosphorus	beans fruits nuts pumpkin and squash seeds sea vegetables sesame seeds sunflower seeds vegetables whole grains	Builds and maintains bones, teeth, hair, and nervous tissue. Assists cells in absorbing fats and carbohydrates.	800 mg.	1539 mg.
Potassium	beans cabbage chestnuts dried fruits dulse fruits kelp leafy greens nuts vegetables	Maintains mineral balance and weight. Tones muscles. Aids disposition, promotes beauty.	—	3666 mg.
Sodium	cucumbers horseradish leafy greens miso root vegetables sea vegetables sesame tamari	Aids digestion, speeds elimination of carbon dioxide, and regulates body fluids and heart action.		2560 mg.

Table 6.3   Mineral Content of Various Sea Vegetables
(milligrams per 100 grams)

Sea Vegetable	Calcium	Phosphorus	Iron	Sodium	Potassium
Agar-agar	567	22	6.3	—	—
Arame	1170	150	12.0	—	*
Dulse	296	267	—	2085	8060
Hijiki	1400	56	29.0	—	*
Irish moss	885	157	8.9	2892	2844
Kelp	1093	240	—	3007	5273
Kombu	800	150	—	2500	*
Nori	260	510	12.0	600	*
Wakame	1300	260	13.0	2500	*

Sources: United States Department of Agriculture and Japan Nutritionist
    Association.

Note: A dash signifies a lack of reliable data for a mineral believed to be present
    in a measurable amount. An asterisk (*) signifies that information is
    not available.

Up From Hypoglycemia— A Case History

Diane Sacolick's Story

Before I became very ill in December of 1982, I had several chronic health problems which I had accepted as a part of my life. The only efforts I made to improve my situation were to see doctors and have prescriptions filled. I was constipated most of the time, usually had a yeast infection, and had between three and six colds a year. I used the laxative Metamucil for constipation, tube after tube of the fungicidal cream Monistat for yeast infections, and antibiotics for colds.

Every year my bladder infections would increase in number and discomfort. After I saw three different doctors and tried eight different drugs, a urologist told me my peri-urethral glands were also infected. His only suggestion was an operation which he said would be extremely painful and probably wouldn't help much. I decided to pass on the operation, and convinced my internist to give me Macrodantin, a medication which had worked for a friend who had similar problems. The Macrodantin stopped the infections and the acute pain, and I took it daily as preventive medicine.

I needed to take Motrin, an anti-inflammatory, every four hours during my period or else, by the time four and a half hours were up, I'd be in tears from the pain in my abdomen. Even with the medication, I was uncomfortable and severely depressed during my period and found it very difficult to get through the day.

I came to Washington, DC in August, 1982 to attend Georgetown Law School. My body endured lack of sleep and poor eating habits remarkably well until October. Then I started to have occasional dizzy spells. I'd become depressed without having the faintest idea why. I came down with a cold that wouldn't go away and was bedridden for two one-week periods, sleeping up to twenty hours some days. The dizzy spells began to come more and more frequently, now accompanied by difficulty in breathing, blurred vision, and tears. The only advice doctors or nurses gave me at this time was to "take it easy," and one gave me a prescription for antibiotics. My throat, sinuses, ears, and nose were all infected at one point.

By December, I was unable to read and study for exams, so I deferred them until January. I went home to Manhattan. My family doctor could not find anything wrong with me.

At this point, I was so depressed that I started contemplating suicide. Since there was nothing wrong with me physically, according to the doctor, I thought I must be going crazy. I considered checking into a mental hospital, but I continued searching for an answer.

While I was home my mother had a party and I met a woman there who had been diagnosed as hypoglycemic. She had some of the same problems. This was it! I thought. I took a Glucose Tolerance Test a few days later. My worst symptoms appeared in full force both during and after the test: dizziness, blurred vision, breathing difficulty, crying spells. The doctors concurred in their diagnosis of my condition as hypoglycemia.

In early January I started the diet standardly prescribed for hypoglycemia by physicians—high in protein, low in carbohydrate. My daily fare consisted of six to eight small meals which included one of the following foods: milk, cheese, nuts, fish, chicken, red meat, or eggs. I drowned my fish, chicken, and eggs in butter because I loved the taste of it, and because a high-fat diet was supposed to be good for hypoglycemia according to several books I had read. The rest of my diet consisted of low-carbohydrate vegetables such as mushrooms and lettuce. I completely gave up my large intake of cigarettes, coffee, alcohol, diet soda, sugar, flour, and fruit at this time. I notified Georgetown Law School that I would not be returning.

My condition improved somewhat. The depression lifted a bit and dizzy spells came less frequently. Yet, although I was very strict on this diet, I still experienced very severe hypoglycemic symptoms at times. My mind was so clouded that I would constantly forget what I was going to say or where I put something. Many days I would just buy food and prepare my meals; this alone would exhaust me for the whole day. My fingers always had at least two bandages on them, sometimes three or four, as I burned and cut myself many times while cooking. I became afraid to walk outside by myself, afraid that I would collapse in the street. I stayed home most of the time and "gave it time." I gained ten pounds.

By early March I decided something more had to be done. I began a series of visits to an allergist. At his instruction, I recorded everthing I ate and when I ate it for a week; I also noted what my symptoms were and when I experienced them. I wrote down what every object in my apartment was made of, as well as the name of every cosmetic and cleaning item I used. I spent hundreds of dollars on various tests, hundreds more on subsequent appointments.

Over the course of five weeks, I was diagnosed as having other problems besides hypoglycemia, including *Candida albicans* (yeast syndrome), an acute allergic state, inhalant and chemical sensitivities, immune deficiency state, an allergy to milk and milk products, and insufficient pancreatic enzymes and hydrochloric acid. I stopped consuming all milk products. With every meal, I took digestive aids such as hydrochloric acid and Kal-n-zyme." I bought nystatin, a fungicide, to combat the yeast problem, and purchased ten bottles of vitamins to boot. I felt much better, but still had very low energy and suffered occasional "attacks" of dizziness accompanied by breathing and vision difficulty.

I was not very comfortable with my new regime, and the next step was expensive allergy testing and rotating foods, which involves eating no one food more than once every four days. I knew this wasn't going to help me and couldn't bear the thought of doing it. When the allergist's assistant suggested that I remove all the plants from my apartment—as mold on them was suspected of causing my symptoms—I knew there had to be a better solution. My diet became more and more restricted and boring as I tried to figure out what was making me sick.

About this time, the Hypoglycemia Association, Inc. of Maryland sent me a bulletin which included a description of the next meeting. Bill and Barbara Taylor were going to speak to H.A.I. about macrobiotics. It appealed to me instantly. I was so sick of red meat and chicken. I read Dr. Sattilaro's book, *Recalled by Life,* and became very excited because I strongly sensed macrobiotics was going to help me.

After hearing the Taylors speak, I was more than ready to begin exploring macrobiotics. I made an appointment with Michael Rossoff, a macrobiotic counselor and acupuncturist in Bethesda, Maryland. After the interview and assessment, he suggested a dietary plan for my condition. The recommendations were for food, acupressure points and books—not drugs or vitamins.

After three days of following these recommendations, my six months of dizzy spells and accompanying symptoms disappeared, never to return. I was elated. Within seven months of following the macrobiotic diet, most of my other problems also disappeared. I have no allergic reactions, I no longer suffer from constipation, and this is the longest I have gone in years without a cold, yeast infection, or bladder infection. In September of 1983 I had my first period without cramps in six years. This improvement was accelerated by a series of ten acupuncture treatments I received while maintaining my new way of eating.

I have never before eaten such a varied and fun "diet." Both cooking and eating are a great pleasure for me now. Instead of eating every two to three hours, I enjoy three meals a day. I'm no longer a slave to the clock. If I choose to, I can now wake up in the morning, exercise and wait as much as three hours before eating, instead of staggering from my bed to the kitchen. I've also lost the weight I gained earlier this year.

My thinking is clearer, and I am happier, calmer, and more patient than ever before. At times I do get tense and impatient, and I still occasionally have trouble with fatigue, but—all in all—my health is improving much more quickly than I would have ever thought possible.

Another wonderful aspect of macrobiotics is the cost compared to most alternative approaches to better health. Most of the food is inexpensive, especially when compared to meat and cheese. While I was on the high-protein diet I felt so deprived and unhappy that I would often "treat" myself to expensive cheeses and meat. Now there are no tests to take, and no drugs or vitamins to buy.

And, of course, the value of increased energy and happiness experienced through macrobiotics is priceless. ■

By Diane Sacolick. Reprinted by permission of *MacroMuse Magazine*, 4905 Del Ray Avenue, Suite 400, Bethesda, MD 20814. Copyright 1984 (Issue #14).

7

Key Macrobiotic Foods

The macrobiotic diet is in accordance with the latest scientific evidence on diet and nutrition, yet the rich blend of tradition and common sense that lies at its core is perhaps an even better reason to eat macrobiotically. Since the advent of agriculture, about twelve thousand years ago, the majority of humans have eaten a diet consisting of whole grains, whole grain products, vegetables, and beans, with limited quantities of animal foods.

Following the agricultural revolution of the 1800s, the modern diet began to change rapidly. The abundance of inexpensive grain made animal husbandry profitable, and meat and dairy foods became widely available. The invention of the roller mill changed the way bread was made, by refining whole grains—separating the bran and germ portions from the endosperm. The prosperity of the early 1900s provided the average individual with access to refined foods and meats that previously were available only to the wealthy. During the past seventy-five years or so, our food supply has become increasingly artificial, and animal foods have gained in popularity. Macrobiotics favors a more traditional way of eating that emphasizes natural, wholesome foods.

In this chapter and the next, we will discuss the nutritional value, interesting aspects, and uses of macrobiotic foods, beginning with whole grains.

WHOLE GRAINS: OUR SOURCE OF ENERGY

The human physiology has not adjusted well to the new habits of eating "fast foods." There is no better illustration of this fact than the growing interest in whole foods, especially whole grains. Thousands of years ago our ancestors began eating the nutritious fruit and seed combination we call whole grain. Since then, many cultures have adopted grains as their staple food. The ancient Chinese depended upon millet, buckwheat, and rice as their staples; the Aztecs and Mayans subsisted mainly on corn; the Egyptians grew some of the world's finest wheat; the early Europeans relied on wheat, rye, barley, and oats; the Britons, oats and wheat; the Hindus, rice and wheat; and a number of African peoples cultivated millet. Some of our ancestors even worshipped grain as a god of life, the fabric of which humans were made. The Japanese word for "peace and harmony" also denotes the eating of grains.

Whole grains are grains that are eaten intact. In whole grains, none of the edible portions (the bran, germ, and endosperm) are removed. On the macrobiotic diet, whole barley, buckwheat, brown rice, millet, oats, rye, and wheat are pressure-cooked, boiled, or baked into casseroles. Whole grain products, ranging from sourdough whole wheat bread to spaghetti are also eaten. Almost any refined grain product that you can find can also be made from whole grains.

Whole grains are composed of complex carbohydrates, proteins, fats, vitamins, and minerals in ideal proportions for the needs of the human body. The ratio of complex carbohydrates to protein in the macrobiotic diet is about seven to one. Whole grain itself also reflects this ideal balance, providing about seven times more complex carbohydrates than protein. Whole grains are also an excellent source of fiber, B complex vitamins, Vitamin E, and phosphorous (a key mineral and brain food).

Beyond their healthfulness, there is at least one other reason to use plenty of whole grains. Of all foods, they are probably the least expensive, because they are so widely cultivated. They cost less to grow—and to eat, per food value dollar—than red meat, eggs and other dairy products, poultry, or fish. The grains most recommended for regular use are barley, brown rice, buckwheat, corn, millet, oats, and wheat. Table 7.1 provides a more complete list of whole grains and grain products.

Table 7.1   Whole Grains and Grain Products

For Regular Use	For Occasional Use	To Avoid
Whole barley	Buckwheat noodles	Baked goods
Whole buckwheat	(soba)	containing
Whole corn	Corn grits or	dairy products
Whole medium-	cornmeal	Refined grain
grain brown rice	Couscous	cereals
Whole millet	Cracked wheat	White flour
Whole rye	(bulghur)	products
Whole short-grain	Long-grain	Yeasted breads,
brown rice	brown rice	crackers, cakes,
Whole oats	Pounded sweet rice	cookies, and
Whole wheat	cakes (mochi)	so on
Other whole	Puffed wheat	
cereal grains	gluten (fu)	
	Ramen noodles	
	(whole wheat,	
	rice, buckwheat)	
	Rice cakes	
	Rice kayu	
	(porridge) bread	
	Rye flakes	
	Somen (sifted whole	
	wheat noodles)	
	Sourdough whole	
	wheat or rye bread	
	Steel-cut or	
	rolled oats	
	Sweet brown rice	
	Tortillas	
	Udon (whole	
	wheat noodles)	
	Unyeasted whole	
	wheat or rye bread	
	Wheat gluten	
	(seitan)	
	Whole wheat	
	crackers or matzo	
	Whole wheat pasta	

VEGETABLES

The word "vegetable" is derived from a Latin word meaning able to live or grow, vigorous, lively, and full of life. In keeping with their names, vegetables (and sea vegetables) supply the full spectrum of vitamins and minerals we need to live and grow in good health.

Vegetables provide a variety of colors, tastes, and textures to the macrobiotic diet. Cut into different shapes and cooked in a variety of ways, vegetables add freshness and lightness to dishes containing whole grains and beans. In smaller amounts, pickled or raw vegetables are also used.

Home-grown vegetables are best. They are fresh, full of flavor, and free from synthetic fertilizers or sprays. In season, they can be prepared in countless ways, both cooked and raw. At the harvest, when home-grown and local produce is abundant and inexpensive, fresh vegetables can be dried, pickled, or stored in a cold cellar for use through the winter.

In the winter, summer vegetables such as cucumbers and string beans are often shipped from warm areas like Mexico or Florida to colder climates. But these vegetables have lost the flavor natural to the colder environment; they are out of season and out of balance with local physiological needs. It is better to buy vegetables such as winter squash, cabbage, and root vegetables, which are more suited to cooler weather, or to store local vegetables for use during the winter months.

There are more than a hundred edible vegetables, many of which are included in the three main groups of vegetables recommended on the macrobiotic diet—green leafy vegetables, root vegetables, and ground vegetables.

Green Leafy Vegetables

Fresh leafy greens like collards or kale are among the most nutritious foods available. Pound for pound, they provide more vita-

Table 7.2 Vegetables

FOR REGULAR USE

Green and White Leafy Vegetables	Ground Vegetables	Stem/Root Vegetables
Broccoli	Acorn squash	Burdock
Bok choy	Buttercup squash	Carrots
Brussels sprouts	Butternut squash	Daikon
Carrot tops	Cauliflower	Dandelion root
Chinese cabbage	Hubbard squash	Lotus root
Chives	Hokkaido pumpkin	Onions
Collard greens	Pumpkin	Parsnips
Daikon greens		Radishes
Dandelion greens		Rutabagas
Green cabbage		Salsify
Kale		Turnips
Leeks		
Mustard greens		
Parsley		
Radish greens		
Scallions		
Turnip greens		
Watercress		

FOR OCCASIONAL USE

Alfalfa sprouts	Green peas	Romaine lettuce
Bamboo shoots	Iceberg lettuce	Shiitake mushrooms
Bean sprouts	Jerusalem artichokes	Snow peas
Beets	Jinenjo (mountain	String beans
Celery	potatoes)	Summer squash
Corn-on-the-cob	Kohlrabi and greens	Swiss chard
Cucumbers	Mushrooms	Water chestnuts
Endive	Patty pan squash	Yellow wax beans
Escarole	Red cabbage	

TO AVOID

Asparagus	Plantain	Spinach
Avocados	Potatoes	Sweet potatoes
Curly dock	Purslane	Taro (albi)
Eggplant	Red chard	Tomatoes
Fennel	Red peppers	Yams
Ferns	Shepherd's purse	Zucchini
Green peppers	Sorrel	

mins, minerals and proteins than meat does—for a fraction of the cost. If you are not in the habit of eating fresh greens, you can begin by adding them to soups or sautéed vegetables, until you can also enjoy them cooked separately, served with whole grains and beans.

Greens are important to the macrobiotic diet for several reasons. One reason is that they are rich in chlorophyll—a protein compound that aids in creating healthy red blood cells. Leafy greens are also an excellent source of Vitamin C, calcium, and alkaline minerals. These neutralize excess acidity in the blood. One reason it is recommended that fish be eaten along with greens and a little grated raw daikon (white radish) is that the latter two provide vitamins and minerals that help us to digest and use the nutrients in the fish better. Fresh greens enjoy a long growing season and are available locally in many parts of the country all year round.

Root Vegetables

As a group, the root vegetables are a good source of vitamins and minerals, and an excellent supplier of complex carbohydrates. Dense and compact root vegetables such as carrots, rutabagas, and parsnips, are rich in minerals and complex carbohydrates, and, compared to the leafy vegetables, require greater digestive effort. In the process they promote warmth and improve digestion by bringing more blood into the abdominal region. This warming property, and the fact that they can easily be stored in a cold cellar through the winter, makes them an ideal food for the colder months of the year. Moreover, in autumn and winter, they are less expensive than vegetables grown elsewhere and sold out of season.

Ground Vegetables

Nutritionally, ground vegetables such as squash and cabbage fall between the leafy greens and the root vegetables. Like the roots, they are a good source of vitamins and minerals and an excellent supplier of complex carbohydrates. Ground vegetables are good in winter, as they are both warming and filling. In addition, they can satisfy even the sweetest tooth when they are picked ripe and cooked properly.

Vegetables to Avoid

Some vegetables containing irritants and mildly toxic alkaloids (alkaline substances) are listed in Table 7.2 under the heading *To Avoid*. Almost all of these have their origin in the tropics. Tomatoes, asparagus, red chard, beet greens, spinach, and rhubarb are also high in oxalic acid, which inhibits the absorption of calcium in the body, weakening bones and teeth, and possibly leading to kidney stones.

Other vegetables, including zucchini, avocado, eggplant, potato, and various edible weeds, are best avoided because they can have an unhealthful acidifying effect on the blood if they are consumed on a regular basis, especially by those living in the temperate zone.

BEANS AND SEA VEGETABLES

Nutritious Food from the Sea

Extracts of marine algae (sea vegetables) are found in almost every type of prepared food, from ice cream and pudding to salad dressings, cheeses, and bread. In fact any food item that utilizes thickeners or stabilizers probably contains carrageenan, algin or agar—all extracts of sea vegetables. However, eating sea vegetables in the form of additives is worlds away from eating them directly from the sea.

For centuries people all over the world have harvested sea vegetables for use as food. The Chinese, Irish, British, Icelanders, Canadians, Japanese, American Indians, Hawaiians, Koreans, Russians, Eskimos, and South Africans are just a few of the peoples who have traditionally eaten sea vegetables.

Years ago, in Boston, the purple-colored sea vegetable dulse was sold by street vendors. In the maritime provinces of Canada and in Scotland, a thin, crisp snack made from dulse is still served in pubs. The Russians sell a fermented beverage made from sea vegetables, and a canned vegetable combination called sea cabbage, which includes vegetables such as beets and tomatoes, along with sea vegetables. The coastal Irish have used Irish moss and other sea vegetables for centuries, in traditional recipes for breads, pastries, beverages, and gelatins. The Japanese, who probably eat more sea vegetables than any other people, grade their sea vegetables for quality, just as the United States Department of Agriculture grades meat or dairy products.

Sea vegetables are an important component of the macrobiotic diet. As a group they are among the most nutritious foods on earth. For instance, compared to garden vegetables, kelp has one hundred and fifty times more iodine and eight times more magnesium. Dulse is thirty times richer in potassium than bananas are and has two hundred times the potency of beetroot when it comes to iron content. Nori, a brown sea vegetable that is sold in thin rectangular sheets, rivals carrots in Vitamin A and has twice the protein of some meats. Hijiki, a blue-black, spaghetti-like sea vegetable, contains fourteen times more calcium than whole milk. Kombu, a brown-colored sea vegetable sold in strips about twelve inches long, equals sweet corn in phosphorus. Sea vegetables contain Vitamins A, B_1 (thiamine), C, and E, and the all-important B_{12}, an essential compound that is rare in vegetarian diets but is needed by the body for healthy neuromuscular function and blood rich in iron.

As they grow, sea vegetables convert the inorganic minerals in sea water into organic mineral salts that are combined with amino acids—the ideal way for us to get the minerals needed to protect the heart and nourish the hair, nails, skin, blood, muscles, and bones. In fact, since the advent of modern farming techniques and the subsequent decline in the quality of topsoil, including sea vegetables in the diet may be the only way we can ensure getting a healthy supply of trace elements from food. Along with the essential minerals discussed in Chapter 6, trace elements such as cobalt, copper, chromium, fluorine, manganese, molybdenum, selenium, and zinc are needed in small amounts to maintain normal metabolic processes in the body.

Sea vegetables work directly on the blood, alkalizing it if it is too acid, and reducing any excess stores of fat or mucus. A substance called alginic acid, found in the darker sea vegetables such as kombu and wakame, transforms toxic metals in the intestines into harmless salts that are easily eliminated. At McGill University in Montreal (1964), researchers demonstrated the ability of sea vegetables to remove radioactive strontium-90 from the body.

Beyond their obvious healthfulness, sea vegetables can be quite tasty. Newcomers to the macrobiotic diet will find that when sea

Table 7.3 Recommended Sea Vegetables

Agar-agar	Kelp
Arame	Kombu
Dulse	Nori (laver)
Hijiki	Wakame
Irish moss	

vegetables are added to soups and bean dishes, or cooked with fresh vegetables as recommended in the recipes in this book, they accentuate the flavor of the other ingredients.

Beans and Bean Products

For eight thousand years beans have been held in high esteem by cultures all over the world. Since the agricultural revolution of the 1800s, however, they have become less popular in the West, where meat, poultry, and other animal foods have become the primary sources of protein.

Macrobiotics is slowly returning the long-neglected bean to its rightful place on the modern dinner table—along with whole grains. Traditionally, grain-based diets from all over the world have combined grains with beans. In much of Europe, South and Central America, Africa, parts of Asia, and the Middle East, beans and grains are the main sources of protein and carbohydrates.

Modern science has uncovered the reason why this combination works so well: beans and grains are complementary proteins, one providing the amino acids lacking in the other. Together these foods supply most of the protein in the macrobiotic diet.

Since beans are particularly rich in high-quality proteins—that is, proteins that are of vegetable origin, are easy for the body to digest and use, and are supplied without saturated animal fats—they are more healthful than meat. In fact, beans replace meat in most vegetarian meat analogs (substitutes) and in many baby formulas for children who are allergic to milk. Moreover, beans (especially after they are sprouted) also contain fairly good supplies of some vitamins and minerals. Table 7.4 lists some of the beans and bean products that are used in the macrobiotic diet.

Table 7.4   Beans and Bean Products

For Regular Use	For Occasional Use	
Aduki beans	Bean sprouts	Lima beans
Chick peas	Black beans	Navy beans
Green or brown lentils	Black soybeans	Pinto beans
Miso	Black turtle beans	Red lentils
Natto (fermented	Great northern	Soybeans
soybeans)	beans	Split peas
Natural tamari	Kidney beans	Whole dried peas
soy sauce		
Tempeh		
Tofu (bean curd)		

Whereas whole grains function primarily to provide ready energy in the diet, they are also an important source of the amino acids lacking in beans and bean products. The protein supplied by whole grains is high in quality as well.

Soybeans and Soyfoods

While soybeans are higher in fat and protein than any other beans, they are also the most difficult to digest due to an enzyme called the trypsin inhibitor. Soaking, cooking, and fermenting soybeans destroys their trypsin inhibitors, and it is for this reason that these nutritious beans are processed into tofu, natto, tempeh, miso, and the other soyfoods available in natural foods stores.

A major advantage that fermented soyfoods such as tofu and tempeh have over plain-cooked beans and other protein foods are soyfoods' easy-to-digest, quality proteins. Soyfoods are also easy to cook with and taste great in a variety of ways.

The most frequently used soyfoods on the macrobiotic diet are tofu, dried tofu, tempeh, miso, and natural tamari soy sauce. Tofu is processed from soybeans and pressed into cakes. It has served as an important source of protein for over two thousand years in China, and more than one thousand years in Japan. It contains a higher percentage of usable protein than chicken. Tempeh (pronounced *tem'-pay*) consists of soybeans and/or grains bound by a dense, white mold and formed into compact cakes. Like tofu, it is high in protein, low in fat, contains no cholesterol, and has few calories. It is a wonderful food for dieters. In addition, tempeh is one of the richest vegetarian sources of Vitamin B_{12}. Miso and natural tamari soy sauce will be discussed more fully in the next chapter.

Macrobiotics has promoted the use of traditional soy products in the United States. Their current popularity is due in part to America's increasing consciousness of the relationship between diet and health. Nevertheless, while they provide a relatively inexpensive, tasty supply of an excellent quality and versatile protein, it is important for us to remember that soyfoods aren't a panacea for nutritional problems in this country or for world hunger. They are just one element in a wholesome balanced diet. Like any other high-protein food, they should be eaten in moderation.

We need only small amounts of beans and soyfoods at each meal. The ideal ratio between grains and vegetables on the one hand and beans on the other is 7:1. That is, it is best to eat seven times more whole grains and vegetables than beans and bean products. This translates into about four to six ounces of beans or bean products per day.

Soymilk, soy ice cream, soy yogurt, soy mayonnaise, soy cheesecake and other soyfoods are not recommended for everyday consumption on the macrobiotic diet. However, they do make good supplementary foods for children or others who are in the process of switching to a more macrobiotic diet.

ORGANICALLY GROWN FOODS

Organic growers do not use synthetically compounded fertilizers, pesticides, herbicides, or fungicides. Instead they rely on crop rotation, manure, composting of crop residues, and a number of biologically safe measures to control insects, weeds, and other pests. Organically grown foods are more balanced foods, grown on more naturally balanced soil. This balance fosters healthy, balanced people.

8

Supplementary Macrobiotic Foods

In the macrobiotic diet, condiments and seasonings have a greater subtlety than they do in typical modern fare. Condiments and seasonings add color, flavor, and nutrients to macrobiotic foods, and improve their digestibility as well. Because of their varied significance, condiments and seasonings are considered supplementary foods on the macrobiotic diet.

In addition to condiments and seasonings, the supplementary foods include fish and seafood, fruits, beverages, and snacks. Cooking ingredients such as natural sweeteners and unrefined oils are also supplementary foods.

While whole grains, beans, and vegetables are the main components of the macrobiotic diet, the supplementary foods play a major role in the overall balance of the diet and its adaptability to individual needs.

CONDIMENTS AND SEASONINGS

The proper use of condiments and seasonings is an important aspect of the macrobiotic diet. Both seasonings, for use in cooking, and condiments, for table use, are always employed moderately. Table 8.1 lists the various types that are recommended. Because macrobiotic recipes call on certain regular-use seasonings and condiments quite often, we will briefly discuss their properties and uses.

Sea Salt

Most people today use too much salt, perhaps in an unconscious attempt to compensate for the poor nutritional quality of the salt

Table 8.1   Condiments and Seasonings

FOR REGULAR USE		TO AVOID
Condiments	Seasonings	Condiments and Seasonings
Ginger	Brown rice vinegar	All unnatural, artificial,
Gomashio	Ginger	and/or chemically
Grated daikon	Horseradish	processed seasonings
Kelp-sesame salt	Mirin	Apple cider vinegar
Kombu condiment	Miso	Commercial soy sauce
Natural mustard	Natural mustard	Common salt
Nori condiment	Nori condiment	Ginseng
Pickled vegetables	Onions	Gray sea salt
Roasted sea	Parsley	Iodized salt
vegetable powder	Scallions	Mayonnaise
Sauerkraut	Sea salt	Soy margarine
Tekka	Tamari soy sauce	Spices (curry, pepper,
Umeboshi plums	Tekka	cumin, chili, etc.)
or paste	Umeboshi plums	Wine
	or paste	Wine vinegar
	Umeboshi vinegar	

that is widely available, and to counterbalance a high intake of animal protein and fat. The increased consumption of common salt has led to numerous health problems among the general public. If sea salt is used instead of common salt, however, we find that the body becomes stronger and more balanced, and that there are fewer health problems. In macrobiotics, the quality of salt in the diet is as important as the quantity.

Common salt, the salt used in most prepared foods and eaten by most people in this country, is mined from inland salt deposits, heated to extremely high temperatures, and refined. Potassium iodide or sodium iodide is added to common salt to create iodized salt. Dextrose (sugar), sodium bicarbonate, and sodium silico-aluminate are often added to keep the salt white and easy to pour.

Sea salt is obtained by the simple process of concentrating sea water under the sun. It contains more trace minerals, and no additives. Up to 5 percent of sea salt is composed of naturally occuring potassium, calcium, magnesium, and trace elements, which are responsible for the mild flavor and good taste of sea salt. Most importantly, these naturally-occurring minerals and trace elements can be readily assimilated by the body.

Deciding upon the amount of salt to use can be difficult. Depending upon where you live and how much sodium you lose through perspiration, your need for salt will vary. In general, individuals in hotter climates have a slightly greater need for salt, along with an increased need for liquids and unrefined vegetable oils in the diet.

Sea salt is best used in cooking, rather than on the table, because it dissolves more quickly with heat. Gomashio (crushed, toasted sesame seeds mixed with sea salt) is better for table use; the oils, flavor, and minerals in the sesame seeds help balance the raw salt.

The amount of salt in the diet also includes other condiments, such as natural tamari soy sauce and miso, which are about twenty percent good-quality salt.

Miso, Tamari, and Tamari Soy Sauce

Miso is fermented soybean paste made from soybeans, sea salt, and sometimes combinations of whole grains, seasonings, or sea vegetables. Miso is available in many different colors and degrees of saltiness. In addition to being a good source of sodium, it is an excellent source of easily digested protein. In general, miso is rich in live enzymes that aid digestion and promote bowel health.

Good-quality miso that has been naturally fermented is an important ingredient in many recipes, especially soups. It can also be used in bean dishes, salad dressings, condiments, and gravies.

Among natural foods shoppers there remains some confusion between real tamari and tamari soy sauce. Real tamari isn't soy sauce at all, but rather the liquid drained off in the process of making miso. A small amount of real tamari can be used on occasion in place of tamari soy sauce. Real tamari is thicker, stronger in color and flavor, and is slightly more expensive than tamari soy sauce.

Tamari soy sauce is made from soybeans and wheat, without additives or preservatives. Like miso, real tamari and tamari soy sauce are salty-tasting and flavorful. Make sure that the tamari soy sauce you buy is natural, as the ordinary soy sauce sold in supermarkets and many Oriental groceries, and served in restaurants, generally contains corn syrup, artificial coloring, and preservatives.

Brown Rice Vinegar

Brown rice vinegar is simply vinegar made from brown rice. It is used to make salad dressings and relishes. Brown rice vinegar is preferred over wine or cider vinegar because it is less acidic. Nevertheless, it is best to use it in small amounts for flavoring.

Umeboshi

Umeboshi plums are plums pickled in sea salt. These mildly sour and very salty plums may be used whole or in the form of a paste, in cooking or at the table. Umeboshi are highly alkalizing and are used to combat overacidity and stomach upset. They aid in the digestion of foods and promote healthy intestinal flora, as the lactic acid in them is able to neutralize harmful microorganisms. Umeboshi are also helpful in clearing the bowel of putrefaction, thereby reducing gas pains.

Gomashio

Gomashio, or sesame salt, is used as a table condiment. It is made by grinding one part sea salt with ten to sixteen parts toasted whole brown sesame seeds. A mortar and pestle or a Japanese suribachi (a special type of bowl) works well for making sesame salt at home. It can also be purchased in some natural foods stores. A pinch or two of sesame salt on whole grains or vegetables will add to their flavor and digestibility. Table 8.1 lists other table condiments.

A Note on Spices

One important point to remember about the macrobiotic diet is that the foods themselves, enhanced with just a little sea salt, flavor the meals. Black pepper, catsup, mustard, and strong spices, such as cayenne pepper, turmeric, cumin, and curry powder overpower delicately flavored meals and are generally not used on the macrobiotic diet. It is generally best to avoid stimulants (such as ginseng) and aromatic herbs, although they may be used in cooking for special occasions.

Table 8.2   Natural Sweeteners
Recommended for Occasional Use

Amasake	Fresh or cooked fruits
Apple juice or cider	Mirin
Barley malt	Raisins
Chestnuts	Rice malt
Dried temperate-climate fruits	Yinnie (rice) syrup

NATURAL SWEETENERS

All sweeteners are concentrated sugars, and if abused, they tend to affect blood sugar levels and overall health. Sweeteners aren't particularly recommended as a source of nutrition, but moderate amounts of good-quality, natural fruit and vegetable sweeteners are not harmful. Honey, molasses, and so-called "natural sugar" ought to be avoided along with cane and beet sugar (sucrose). The best sweeteners to use are rice syrup and barley malt, which are both made by cooking down grains.

Amasake (rice milk) is a sweetener made by cooking sweet rice and then adding koji, a fermentation starter. After a few hours of fermentation, the rice is cooked again. Mixed with water, amasake can make a sweet milk substitute, or a delicious pudding. It can also be cooked down to make a syrup for sweetening other foods. Regardless of the climate or geographical location, all of the natural sweeteners listed in Table 8.2 can be used moderately.

UNREFINED COOKING OILS

The oils used in macrobiotic cooking are unrefined, unlike commercial oils. Commercial corn oil, for example, is processed by cooking corn in water at a high temperature and then crushing it and treating it with lye and bleach. The oil is reheated in a vacuum for twelve hours to deodorize it. Finally a synthetic antioxidant is added to prevent spoilage. To make margarine, the refined oil is saturated with hydrogen to solidify it. This processing results in inferior-quality fats, which are difficult to digest.

Naturally extracted, unrefined vegetable oils are easier to digest. They also strengthen cell and capillary structure, lubricate the skin and hair, and provide raw materials for the production of lecithin, which plays an important role in lowering blood cholesterol levels. In addition, unrefined vegetable oils contain a natural preservative in the form of Vitamin E.

While a deficiency of fats is virtually impossible on the macrobiotic diet, since most natural foods contain some fat, a shortage of this nutrient can lead to cold hands and feet, stunted growth in children, dermatitis, poor sexual performance, hot flashes, and a lowered resistance to stresses of all kinds. Over the long run, too few fats in the diet could also damage the nervous system.

Oil is similar to salt in that a moderate amount is necessary while a lot can be harmful. A teaspoon of oil per person, used every day or every other day (in cooking) is usually adequate.

Two specific unrefined oils recommended for regular use are corn and sesame oil (light or dark). These are chemically stable and tolerate heat well. Besides corn and sesame oils, small amounts of unrefined sunflower, safflower, soybean, olive, and peanut oils can be used. As Table 8.3 indicates, you should avoid the use of cottonseed oil, palm kernel oil, and cocoa butter (oil made from coconuts). These are less stable and become rancid more easily. Many so-called health food candies, such as the popular carob treats, often use these inferior oils because they are highly saturated and simulate the texture of chocolate.

Table 8.3   Cooking Oils

For Regular Use	For Occasional Use	To Avoid
Corn oil	Olive oil	Butter, margarine,
Sesame oil	Peanut oil	or shortening
(light and dark)	Safflower oil	Lard or other
	Soybean oil	animal fats
	Sunflower oil	Refined, chemically
		processed oils
		Soy margarine

FRESH FISH AND SEAFOODS

The macrobiotic diet for people living in temperate (four-season) climates need not be totally vegetarian; it can include moderate amounts of white-meat fish and certain shellfish. Besides being exposed to fewer chemicals and pollutants than other animal protein sources, fish is nutritionally superior.

Livestock and other animal protein sources cannot be compared with the wild game our ancestors ate because today's animals are fed hormones and antibiotics to artificially fatten them for market. They are also given shelter from the elements and all the food they can eat. This means fattier meat and poorer-quality milk. Not only did our ancestors consume a smaller amount of animal proteins and fats than we do, but what they did eat was better for them.

Meats are often aged for months, and preservatives and red dyes are used to prevent them from turning black and blue. Poultry is also injected with preservatives and dipped in solutions to increase shelf life. Fresh fish, especially freshwater or ocean fish caught locally, is usually eaten within two or three days of the catch. It is generally marketed without added hormones, coloring agents, antibiotics, or preservatives. One exception is freshwater fish (especially trout) bred in fish farms, as they have been fed an unnatural diet and raised in an artificial environment.

Most fish is lower in fat and cholesterol than red meats, milk, eggs, cheese, yogurt, or poultry, and it is generally higher in its percentage of usable protein than any of these as well. It is also easier to digest.

Table 8.4   Fresh Fish and Seafoods

For Regular Use	For Occasional Use	To Avoid
Flounder	Carp	Bluefish
Haddock	Clams	Mackerel
Halibut	Cod	Salmon
Herring	Red snapper	Swordfish
Smelt	Scrod	Tuna
Sole	Shrimp	Other fishes with
Trout	Oysters	red meat or
		blue skin

When eating fish, it is a good idea to increase the amount of vegetables at the meal, especially greens. It is also good to use a garnish
such as several tablespoons of grated raw daikon with a few drops
of tamari. This will help to balance the nutrients in the fish and aid
in its digestion.

Since they are higher in fat and cholesterol, shellfish should be
used less often than white-meat fish. Individual servings of fish and
shellfish can be about four to six ounces, eaten one or two times per
week (if you are in good health). As supplementary foods, fish and
shellfish enhance the macrobiotic diet, but they are not necessary
for balanced nutrition. Table 8.4 lists the varieties of fresh fish and
seafoods that are used, along with the types that are best avoided.

When you shop for fish, find out when and where it was caught.
Whenever possible, follow the reports of water quality in your area,
and do not buy any fish or shellfish, including freshwater fish, from
polluted or contaminated waters.

MACROBIOTIC SNACKS

Snacks are especially good between meals if you are hungry. There
are many tasty natural snacks to choose from.

Roasted seeds and nuts, lightly salted with sea salt or natural
tamari soy sauce, make a delightful snack. As they are rich in fat
and somewhat difficult to digest, it is best to eat them in small
amounts. It is most healthful to limit the use of roasted seeds and

Table 8.5   Macrobiotic Snacks

For Occasional Use		To Avoid
Almonds	Rice cakes	Brazil nuts
Chestnuts	Roasted grains	Cashew nuts
Home-made	and beans	Filberts
popcorn	Sesame seeds	Macadamia nuts
Peanuts	Sunflower seeds	Pistachios
Pecans	Walnuts	
Pumpkin seeds		

nuts to two or three handfuls a week as a snack, with only a small amount more, if desired, used as an ingredient in preparing breads, desserts, or vegetable and grain dishes. Small quantities of nut or seed butters (such as sesame, sunflower, or natural peanut butter) can also be used occasionally.

As Table 8.5 indicates, some other good snacks include rice cakes, popcorn, and the roasted grains and beans available at natural foods grocers.

FRESH AND DRIED FRUITS

Fresh fruit is a delicious addition to the macrobiotic diet. Table 8.6 shows the various temperate and tropical climate fruits.

Table 8.6   Fresh and Dried Fruits

FOR OCCASIONAL USE	TO AVOID
Temperate climate fruits	Tropical fruits and juices
Apples	Avocados
Apricots	Bananas
Blackberries	Coconuts
Blueberries	Dates
Cantaloupe	Figs
Cherries	Grapefruits
Cranberries	Guavas
Currants	Kiwis
Grapes	Lemons
Honeydew melon	Limes
Peaches	Mangoes
Pears	Oranges
Plums	Papayas
Prunes	Pineapples
Raspberries	
Raisins	
Strawberries	
Tangerines	
Watermelon	

Fruits that are unripe, those grown out of season and shipped to the winter zone, and tropical fruits are not recommended for people living in the temperate climate zone. However, a healthy individual living in a tropical area may use small amounts of tropical fruits as they become available in season.

Fruits that have been sprayed or chemically treated in any way are best avoided. Local, unsprayed fruits (in season), and dried fruits such as raisins, prunes, apples, pears, apricots, cherries, and currants are recommended. These are best eaten cooked, with a pinch of sea salt if desired, or dried. Upon occasion, fresh, uncooked fruits may be eaten. Since so many fruits are picked unripe, sold out of season, or sprayed with pesticides, it is best to limit fruit consumption to a few servings per week.

BEVERAGES

The beverages most commonly consumed in America are soft drinks, orange juice, tea, coffee, beer, wine, whiskey, and milk. But lately many of these have been linked to a number of health problems. Tea, coffee and colas have been implicated for their caffeine content; flavored soft drinks and juices for their sugar and additives; orange juice due to allergic reactions reported by users, and its acidity; commercial beers and alcoholic beverages for their additives, preservatives, and alcohol; and milk for its cholesterol and fat. In place of these drinks the macrobiotic diet uses a variety of special teas, coffee substitutes, and occasionally fresh juices and other beverages. These are listed in Table 8.7.

Tea, especially twig or stem (bancha) tea, is a healthful and satisfying beverage that can be enjoyed warm or cool. Many varieties of tea, including bancha, come from the plant known botanically as *Camellia sinensis*, which is cultivated in different parts of the world. But teas from this plant vary widely. When and where the plants are grown and harvested, and which parts of the plant are used, determine the strength and caffeine content of the tea. Teas made from young leaves and buds (sold in many gourmet shops) are the most stimulating. Next comes black teas, the most commonly used teas. Both of these types are too stimulating for daily use.

Table 8.7   Beverages

For Regular Use	For Occasional Use	For Less Frequent Use	To Avoid
Amasake	Dandelion tea	Apple juice	Alcohol
Bancha tea	Grain coffee	or cider	Black tea
Roasted barley	Kombu tea	Barley green	Coffee
tea	Mu tea	tea	Commercial
Roasted rice		Fruit juice	beers
tea		(temperate	Decaffeinated
Spring or		climate)	coffee
well water		Green tea	Distilled water
		Naturally	Herb teas (mint,
		fermented	rose hips, etc.)
		beer	Juice drinks
		Sake (rice	(commercial)
		wine)	Municipal or
		Seed/nut milk	tap water
		Vegetable	Soft drinks and
		juice	artificially
			flavored
			bevrages
			Wine

The teas used on the macrobiotic diet are different. Whereas some of them may contain minute quantities of caffeine, they are not processed to increase their caffeine content. Processed brands, which are high in caffeine, are best avoided.

Other teas (not made from the tea plant) recommended for use on the macrobiotic diet are roasted barley or rice tea, dandelion root tea, kombu tea (from kombu sea vegetable), and umeboshi tea (from salted plums). In addition, you may use mu tea, which is an especially strengthening blend of traditional non-stimulating herbs. Other aromatic or medicinal herb teas, such as peppermint, rose hips, or camomile are not recommended. Herbs should be treated as medicine; to use them indiscriminately could be harmful.

All of the beverages mentioned above can be used as a substitute for coffee, but if a more robust flavor is desired, grain coffee made from a blend of roasted grains (with or without chicory root) can be used on occasion. All hot teas and beverages are best made with pure spring or well water, as municipal water supplies may be contaminated with harmful substances such as chlorine or sodium fluoride.

USING SUPPLEMENTARY FOODS

Supplementary foods may make up as much as ten percent of the macrobiotic diet, depending upon your individual tastes and nutritional needs. As a group, the supplementary foods are the most flexible part of the diet. Chapter 12 discusses some of the ways in which the diet may be modified.

People with specific questions regarding modifications of the standard diet are advised to seek the guidance of experienced macrobiotic counselors, but in general those in good overall health may enjoy moderate amounts of the supplementary foods discussed in this chapter.

9

Yin and Yang

Everything in the universe is constantly changing. Each day we experience the result of this unceasing motion as night changes into day, activity changes into rest, youth into old age, life into death, and death into rebirth. An understanding of the changes that govern our lives and the natural environment, and a recognition of the interrelationship between opposite, yet complementary tendencies within these changes, helps us to achieve harmony in our bodies and minds.

The principle of yin and yang is the philosophical foundation of macrobiotics. The way to practice this universal principle in daily life was taught by Lao Tzu, Confucius, Buddha, Moses, Jesus, Muhammed, and other great teachers throughout history. To understand this simple principle and then to live its basic laws is the greatest way to perfect health and long life.

The principle of yin and yang is also known as the Unifying Principle because it states that antagonistic forces complement and unify each other. A clear example of this is man and woman. Though men and women are opposites in many ways, they depend on each other for continued existence. Together they form a unity, each acquiring aspects of the other.

Many different interpretations have been given to yin and yang throughout history. Several thousand years ago in China, for example, the universal process of change was called the Tao. The Taoists and others based their teachings on the underlying principle of yin and yang. In the Hindu religion, Brahman, the absolute, becomes Shiva and Parvati, the god and goddess whose cosmic dance gives rise to all phenomena in the universe. Similarly, in the Shinto religion, Ame-nominakanushi, who stands for infinity, becomes

Takami-musabi and Kami-musubi, the gods of centrifugality and centripetality, from whom the phenomenal universe arises.

In the West, the underlying principle of yin and yang has been expressed in countless ways by various philosophers and teachers. For example, the ancient Greek philosopher Empedocles viewed the universe as an eternal playground of two opposite, yet complementary forces, which he called love and strife. Another classical philosopher, Heraclitus, referring to the eternal process of change as Logos, taught of the opposite, yet complementary nature of all phenomena.

In Judaism, the principle of complementary opposites is expressed in the symbol of the six-pointed Star of David, showing the balanced intersection of descending and ascending triangles. More recently, key ideas in the works of writers and philosophers such as Emerson, Thoreau, Hegel, and Walter Russell, have expressed the underlying principle of yin and yang, while a more natural way of life, based on balance, has been advocated by many thinkers, including Edward Carpenter, Samuel Butler, and George Bernard Shaw.

YIN AND YANG IN MACROBIOTICS

Macrobiotics focuses on the dynamics of yin and yang in daily life. Yin is the name given to energy or movement that has a centrifugal or outward direction, and results in expansion. Thus diffusion, dispersion, expansion, and separation are all yin tendencies. Yang, on the other hand, denotes energy or movement that has a centripetal or inward direction, and results in contraction. Fusion, gathering, contraction, and organization are yang tendencies.

The forces of yin and yang are the most basic and primary, and are found throughout creation. All movement, formation, change, and interaction can be understood in terms of a basic yin and yang equation.

By looking at which of these energies predominate in plants, foods, or individuals, we can classify them as more yin or more yang. However, since all things are relative, nothing is ever completely yin or yang. From an understanding of yin and yang tendencies, we can learn ways to achieve natural harmony and balance in the body and in life.

In the world around us, the sun, daytime, heat and summer all display yang tendencies, while the moon, night, cold, and winter reflect more yin qualities. In the human body we can see the action of both yin and yang in the expansion and contraction of the lungs and heart, or in the stomach and intestines during digestion. Being active, animals (including humans) are more yang than plants, which are stationary. As the following table suggests, there are a number of factors that can be used to determine yin or yang qualities.

Table 9.1   Examples of Yin and Yang

Characteristic	(∇) Yin	(△) Yang
Atomic particle	electron	proton
Attitude	more gentle, passive	more aggressive, active
Biological	more vegetable quality	more animal quality
Climate	temperate, colder	tropical, warmer
Direction	ascent; vertical; outward	descent; horizontal; inward
Flavor	sweet	salty
Food preparation	less cooked	more cooked
Form	longer, thinner	shorter, thicker
Function	diffusion	fusion
Humidity	more wet	more dry
Light	darker	brighter
Movement	more inactive; slower	more active; faster
Nerves	peripheral, orthosympathetic	central, para-sympathetic
Organ structure	more hollow, expansive	more dense, compacted
Position	more outward, peripheral	more inward, central
Sex	female	male
Shape	more expansive	more contracted
Size	larger	smaller
Temperature	colder	hotter
Tendency	expansion	contraction
Texture	softer	harder
Vibration	shorter wave, higher frequency	longer wave, lower frequency
Weight	lighter	heavier
Work	More psychological, mental	More physical, social

YIN AND YANG IN FOODS

Watery, cooling, yin plant foods grow in hot yang climates, while denser, hardier, more yang plant foods grow in temperate, more yin climates. When we begin to realize that our food affects our ability to adapt to local climates and conditions, the importance of balance becomes more clear. All of us follow our natural instincts to some extent in order to maintain balance. When it is cold we turn up the heat. When it becomes warm we seek refreshment. The summer brings lighter eating and less cooking, the winter heavier eating and more thorough cooking. Macrobiotics helps us to become more aware of our intuitive needs for foods well suited to our local environment. It also tells us how to cook and prepare these foods in harmony with our immediate needs and conditions.

Red meat, poultry, hard cheeses, and eggs are more yang than plants. They are the result of a concentration of plants eaten by an animal.

A further division into yin and yang characteristics can be made within the plant kingdom itself. A northern pine, for example, has short, hard needles, while the southern pine develops larger, longer, and softer ones. Root vegetables and seeds are more yang than leaves and branches. Above-the-ground-vegetables such as winter squashes or pumpkins are more yang—more dense and less watery—than tree fruits. In general, plants that grow quickly in warm climates or hot weather, and those that have a higher water content, are more yin. Tropical fruits like papayas, mangoes, avocados, bananas, and citrus fruits, and tropical vegetables such as potatoes, tomatoes, spinach, zucchini, eggplant, and yams are all yin compared with the more hardy plants of northern origin. In the temperate north, indigenous fruits, grains, vegetables, seeds, beans and nuts are smaller, grow more slowly, contain less liquid, and are more yang.

The following chart lists from top (yin) to bottom (yang) and right (yin) to left (yang) many foods commonly eaten on the macrobiotic diet and in many parts of the world.

Within each category of foods listed on the chart, there are yin and yang variations. For example, among the grains, buckwheat (the most yang) thrives in cold climates and in the mountains. Corn (the most yin) likes hot summer weather and grows well in the

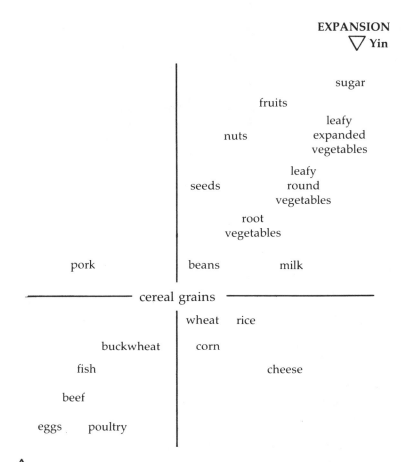

Figure 9.1   General Yin (▽) and Yang (△)
Categorizations of Foods

tropics. Brown rice is in between. Relatively small beans such as aduki are more yang than Lima and soybeans, which are larger and contain more fat and oil. The same is true for nuts and seeds—the smaller and less oily they are, the more yang. Sesame seeds, which are hard and small, are more yang than larger and more oily Brazil nuts or walnuts. Swordfish, salmon, bluefish, mackerel, or tuna (all faster, larger, and more powerful fish) are more yang than smaller white-meat fish such as flounder or sole. Table 9.2 lists the general yin and yang variations of the foods by food category.

Table 9.2   Variations in Yin and Yang by Food Category

	Category	(△) Yang ⟵⟶ (▽) Yin	
Yin ↑	sugar	raw	refined
	fruits	smaller	larger
		growing on ground	growing on tree
		colder climate	warmer climate
	nuts	less oily	more oily
	leafy expanded vegetables	smaller	larger
		growing in colder climate	growing in warmer climate
	seeds	smaller	larger
	leafy round vegetables	smaller	larger
	root vegetables	smaller	larger
	pork	less fatty	more fatty
	beans	small	large
	milk	less fatty	more fatty
	cereal grains	growing in colder climate	growing in warmer climate
	fish	faster-moving	slower-moving
		smaller	larger
	beef	drier	more fatty
	cheese	more condensed	less condensed
		less fatty; saltier	more fatty; sweeter
	eggs	smaller	larger
↓ **Yang**	poultry	smaller	larger
		high-flying	low-flying

The macrobiotic diet is made up of foods located in the center of Figure 9.1: the foods that are most balanced in terms of yin and yang and in nutritional factors for adults in a temperate climate. Chapter 12, Balancing the Macrobiotic Diet, discusses the practical application of the workings of yin and yang in cooking and eating.

When we eat foods out of harmony with our bodily needs, such as meats, eggs, and hard salty cheeses (all yang), we create an equal and opposite craving for sugar, strong or stimulating spices, herbs, or condiments, coffee, alcohol, ice cream, and tropical fruits (all yin), in an attempt to balance our physical and mental condition. The swings from one extreme to the other can destroy the foundation of good health and lead to disease.

All physical and mental imbalances can be explained as being caused by excessive yin, excessive yang, or a combination of excessive yin and yang in food choice, attitude, and lifestyle. An example of a symptom arising from excess yin is a headache caused when the cells and tissues of the brain expand due to an overindulgence in alcohol. A headache caused by excess yang, on the other hand, arises when the cells and tissues of the brain contract and press against each other, causing pain. This example shows that seemingly similar symptoms can arise from opposite causes. It also explains why aspirin (extreme yin) can relieve some headaches (ones due to yang causes), while it is powerless to relieve a headache due to a hangover (an excess yin cause).

Many factors are weighed by the trained macrobiotic counselor in determining a person's overall condition and the best diet for that person. Nevertheless, the macrobiotic diet for healing usually involves a combination of whole grains, vegetables, beans, and supplementary foods—the standard diet outlined in this book—adapted to suit the individual's needs.

Beyond the purely physical effects of extreme yin or yang foods and lifestyles, these imbalances have a profound impact on a person's psyche as well.

THE BIGGER THE FRONT THE BIGGER THE BACK

In everything there is a front and a back. Macrobiotic theory suggests that the bigger the front, the bigger the back will be. For example, the huge military arms race and its implications for the future survival of human life (*the front*) has also created a global desire for world peace (*the back*).

Modern society's tendency to take a symptomatic approach to illness *(the front)* has created an inspiring revolution in health care called the wholistic approach *(the back)*.

Our sedentary lifestyle and questionable habits *(the front)* have created a rapidly expanding natural foods industry interested in improving the quality of our nutrition, and widespread interest in fitness *(the back)*.

10

The Joy of Exercise

Walking, our natural means of transport, is an excellent form of exercise. Other exercises are used to produce specific results, as every individual has specific exercise needs. The exercise program we suggest, combined with the macrobiotic diet and a busy and active life, will improve cardiovascular health and normalize the flow of energy in the body.

The routine offers the same positive results as many common exercise programs such as calisthenics, weight training, and aerobics. The benefits are increased flexibility, endurance, and muscle tone; healthier blood; and weight loss. But the exercises presented here are superior because they work on all the major body systems rather than on a select few. Actually, the real focus of these exercises is on the internal workings of the body—the glands, organs, and overall metabolism. They are adapted from the centuries-old practice of *do-in*, a form of exercise and self-massage that promotes rejuvenation and longevity.

Many exercise programs concentrate on the external muscles while any internal benefits are secondary. You will certainly shape up performing the exercises that follow, but more importantly, you will be balancing and normalizing the flow of energy inside your body. In addition, you will be recharging your nervous system and your body's energy focal point located just below the navel. As this center of energy becomes charged your level of physical and mental energy will surge.

After just a few weeks of daily exercise, your breathing will be freer, your muscles will become more toned, you will have more energy, and your appetite for more wholesome foods will increase.

The stretching movements will add flexibility and strength, and at the same time help you to develop the capacity for deep muscle relaxation. In time, your posture will also improve, your need for sleep will decrease, and your physical endurance and powers of concentration will increase. In other words, you will begin to experience what health really is—the joy of being alive and well.

By improving breathing capacity and circulation, exercise helps cleanse the blood. The added oxygen in the blood oxidizes (burns) impurities, and the lymphatic system, which carries wastes from the cells, also cleanses itself.

The added oxygen intake from exercise stimulates an increase in the basal metabolic rate, the rate at which the body uses energy when at rest. An increase in basal metabolic rate, along with increased activity, is an important factor in controlling weight, as it means that the body is burning food energy (calories) more rapidly.

Whether you begin the exercises when you are healthy or unwell, you will probably start to notice improvements after the first few sessions. *It is important, however, not to overdo it in the beginning, especially if you haven't exercised in some time.* To minimize the risk of your overdoing the exercises presented here, we suggest a one-minute rest period between each exercise. If you are not sure how much exercise is too much, try shortened movements and lengthened rest pauses between exercises. Don't extend your body beyond its present limits by holding on to your legs or feet if this causes pain. The movements aren't a test of flexibility, but rather a way to gradually improve it.

Check with your physician before beginning any exercise program if you have a history of heart problems or other physical restrictions. If you experience any sudden pains, cramps, or aches, slow down or stop exercising until they go away.

If you are confined to a wheelchair or to bed, even gentle or subtle movements may aid your body's healing efforts.

MERIDIAN STRETCHES

The following exercise routine will take between twenty and forty minutes to perform depending upon your energy level and desire. Its primary emphasis is upon the system of meridians described by modern acupuncture theory. There are fourteen meridians (lines of energy flow) which run up and down the body, extending to both internal organs and external body parts, including the toes, hands, face, and scalp. According to Oriental medicine, if the electromagnetic energy flow through the meridians is harmonious and free, the person is healthy. The meridian stretches help re-establish and maintain a balanced energy flow. While performing the routine, imagine clear and unblocked energy flowing through each meridian as described in the captions beneath Figures 10.1 through 10.7. Such positive mental focus will enhance the effectiveness of the stretches.

Use the routine once a day, in the morning or evening, or whenever you can find the time. Keep in mind that it is better to do the exercises every other day than it is to miss several days in a row.

When exercising, hold each of the positions at their point of extension for one full breath, then revert to the original position, and rest for about thirty seconds before moving onto the next stretching movement. Also, in all of the movements, bend from the waist rather than from your upper back. The point of extension will be different for each person; the distance you can stretch is not nearly so important as performing the exercise with correct form.

When you complete an exercise, *be sure to pause for the full minute before moving on to the next exercise.* In a twenty-minute routine, this will cut the actual exercise time to about fifteen minutes—with five minutes of rest to allow your body to prepare for the next exercise. The exercises are illustrated in Figures 10.1 through 10.7.

Trunk Bend

Standing, with your feet shoulders' width apart, clasp your hands behind your back. Slowly bend forward, raising your arms behind you and keeping the hands clasped. Bend from the waist as far forward and as far down as possible, extending the hands beyond the line of the head, as shown in Figure 10.1. Take a full breath and slowly return to the original standing position. Pause briefly and repeat the movement, a dozen times in all. Rest for a minute and move to the next exercise.

(a) starting position   (b) extension

Figure 10.1   Trunk Bend
This exercise stimulates the lung and large intestine meridians, which run along the outside of the arm and hand.

Alternate Leg Stretch

Sit with both legs extended in front of you, opened as widely as possible. Reach forward with both arms extended toward your right foot, making sure the knees are locked with the backs of the legs close to or touching the floor. As shown in Figure 10.2, bend the entire trunk of your body from the waist, letting your head drop as you stretch. When you reach the point of extension take a full breath. Slowly return to the original sitting position. Turn and repeat the same movement toward the opposite leg. Pause for a breath before repeating. Keep alternating until you have stretched in each direction six times. Stand and rest for a minute, and move on to the next exercise.

Figure 10.2   Alternate Leg Stretch
This exercise stimulates the liver and gall bladder meridians. The liver meridian runs along the inside of the leg to the torso. The gall bladder meridian passes along the leg, over the torso, under the arm from front to back, and over the shoulder, extending up to the temple.

Front Body Stretch

Sit on the floor with your legs folded to the sides as shown in Figure 10.3, and place a pillow or two behind your buttocks. Slowly and carefully bend backwards, lowering your shoulders and back to the floor. If this is too difficult, fold your arms behind and underneath for support. With shoulders and back on the floor, extend both arms above the head. In the extended posture take seven full breaths while concentrating on the energy flow through the meridians. Return to a standing position and rest for one minute before moving to the next exercise. Eventually you will become able to do this stretch without your arms for support and without the aid of the pillows.

(a) viewed from above;
arms used for support

(b) viewed from above;
arms overhead

(c) side view

Figure 10.3   Front Body Stretch
This exercise stimulates the stomach meridian and the spleen-pancreas meridian. The stomach meridian runs up the front of the leg, across the torso, ending on the face, and the spleen/pancreas meridian runs up the inside of the leg and over the chest, ending under the arm.

Double Leg Stretch

Sit on the floor with your legs together and extended straight in front of you. Bending forward from the waist, reach with your hands toward the toes of both feet. Make sure your knees remain locked and the backs of your legs rest against the floor. At the point of extension, which is illustrated in Figure 10.4, take one full breath and slowly return to the original sitting position. Pause briefly and repeat until you have performed a dozen stretches. Stand and rest for a minute before going to the next exercise.

Figure 10.4 Double Leg Stretch

This exercise stimulates the kidney and bladder meridians. The kidney meridian runs up the back of the leg and around the body, ending on the chest. The bladder meridian runs down the back of the torso and leg.

(a) starting position   (b) extension

Figure 10.5   Open Leg Bend

This exercise stimulates the heart and small intestine meridians. The heart meridian runs up the arm, ending under the armpit, and the small intestine meridian runs up the back of the arm, ending on the face.

Open Leg Bend

Sit on the floor with your legs open in front of you, soles of the feet together, and knees wide apart. Holding your toes with both hands, slowly bend forward from the waist, bringing your nose toward the arches of the feet (see Figure 10.5). At the point of extension, take a full breath and return to the original sitting position. Pause briefly and repeat until you have performed a dozen bends. Stand and rest for a minute before moving to the next exercise.

Crossover Bend

Sit on the floor with your ankles crossed close to the body and knees wide apart. Also cross your arms in front so that the right hand grasps the left knee, and the left hand the right knee. Now bend forward from the waist as far as you can, trying to touch your forehead to the floor in front of you. At the point of extension, which is illustrated in Figure 10.6, take a full breath and return to the original cross-legged sitting position. Pause briefly and repeat until you have performed twelve stretches. Stand and rest for a minute before going to the side stretch.

(a) starting position   **(b) extension**

Figure 10.6   Crossover Bend
This exercise stimulates the two comprehensive circulatory meridians, which are known as the triple heater (TH) and the governing vessel (GV). The TH runs along the middle of the inside and outside of the arm; the GV passes up and down the front and back of the torso from the groin to the buttocks.

Side Stretch

Stand with feet at the width of one and a half shoulders apart, hands extended straight above your head, and thumbs (but not hands) clasped together. Bend from the waist to the right side until your trunk and arms are at a ninety-degree angle to the floor, as shown in Figure 10.7. At the point of extension, twist your trunk so that you are now looking towards the ground, keeping thumbs clasped and arms extended outward as far as possible. Hold the position for a full breath. Rotate the trunk again, slowly returning to the original position. Pause and repeat the exercise to the left side, and then alternate right and left sides until you have performed the movement six times on each side.

(b) extension

(a) starting position

(c) twisting

Figure 10.7   Side Stretch

This exercise stimulates many of the meridians simultaneously.

WALKING

Many people have begun to jog or run over the last few years. Perhaps one reason why jogging has become so popular is that it balances a high-fat diet. It helps to develop extra routes of circulation for blood to flow through, while a high-fat, high-cholesterol diet tends to close normal routes off. So jogging or running increases circulatory capacity and may reduce the risks associated with eating the modern diet.

Unfortunately, jogging has drawbacks, too. While over a period of time it may be a balancing form of exercise for the heart and circulation, in the short run it tends to unevenly stress the heart and other body parts and systems. Although some people can enjoy jogging or running, joggers are frequently halted by back problems, bone and joint disorders, and kidney damage, due to the shock of pounding up and down while running.

In the words of Thomas Jefferson, "The sovereign invigorator of the body is exercise, and of all the exercises walking is best." The rewards of just plain walking equal those that can be obtained from any other exercise, with half the risk of injury or exhaustion.

If you are like many people today, however, you can probably think of at least five reasons why you couldn't put this book down right this minute and take a walk: it's too dark out, there's no place to walk, there isn't time, it's raining, it's cold, and so on. It is easy to make excuses, but you can't get the benefits of an exercise program by reading about it. You have to do it. Safety is always a consideration, but during the day parks and schoolyards are generally good places for a refreshing walk. If it's raining, put on a raincoat and a pair of boots and bring an umbrella. If it's cold, wear a coat and a hat. A half hour of walking per day helps to:

- Control your weight, by increasing basal metabolic rate
- Improve blood circulation and quality, warming the hands and feet
- Prevent heart problems and other illnesses
- Aid digestion and elimination
- Act as a mild appetite suppressant

• Keep bones healthy and strong

• Relieve tensions and worry

• Prevent respiratory disorders

• Burn off fat

• Tone muscles, especially thighs, calves, and hips

• Improve looks.

Some exercise physiologists consider walking to be a "second heart" because during walking the muscles of the feet, calves, thighs, buttocks, and abdomen rhythmically contract and release. So does the diaphragm, the powerful muscle that is part of our breathing apparatus. As the muscles contract and release they squeeze the veins, pressing the blood upwards towards the heart.

When you do not walk, your blood tends to pool in the belly, hips, thighs, and feet. Circulation slows, and the heart must work harder to make sure that enough oxygen reaches the cells and that wastes are removed. When you stand still or sit for long periods of time, your brain also suffers from a lack of oxygen.

To begin a walking program, all you need is a comfortable pair of shoes. Running shoes are especially good. For maximum benefit, your stride should be brisk. Let your arms swing freely at your sides and keep your head up. Rhythm is the key.

Try to find a place to walk where you can establish a steady pace without a lot of starts and stops. If possible, avoid crowded sidewalks and noisy or heavily trafficked avenues, and find a park, a trail in the woods, or a beach. Walking barefoot on the grass or on a beach is the most invigorating of all.

SOME ADDITIONAL TIPS

Make it a priority to walk every day, for it is important to make time to do the things that will benefit your health.

The morning is the best time to walk. Many of the most confident, relaxed, and content people have learned to begin their day with light exercise and a walk. The air seems fresher and the activity seems to awaken and stimulate physical and mental processes which otherwise remain half asleep. Scientists explain this phenomenon by pointing to endorphins, chemicals that are released inside us by physical activities such as a good walk. If scientists have discovered anything that could be called "happy" chemicals, they would be the endorphins. A brisk morning walk is much better than a cup of coffee for "starting your engine."

It will benefit your health and the environment if you start your *own* engine instead of driving your car for every little errand. When you must drive, park in the space farthest from the store rather than the closest. Walk to work. Get a dog and let him walk you if you won't take yourself out. As long as you stay warm and dry, a walk in rain or snow will leave you feeling vitalized.

A half hour each day is a good amount of time to spend walking. A full hour every other day is also fine. Whatever you do, don't overdo it. Especially if you are ill, convalescent, or out of shape, start out slowly, walking no more than is comfortable. Every few days increase the distance by 10–20 percent.

Ideally, before you head out to walk, perform either the stretches presented in this chapter or other light stretching exercises. If you feel too stiff and a little sleepy in the morning, get out and walk first and do the stretches when you return. Follow your morning exercise session with one of the macrobiotic breakfast dishes in the recipe section.

Walking and stretching, together with a wholesome diet, are important aspects of the macrobiotic way. Many people have found health and happiness in these simple principles.

11

Improving the Quality of Life

By becoming more aware of the factors that affect the quality of life, we can improve it. So far we have discussed the roles of diet and exercise in improving physical health. In this chapter we will discuss the effects of diet, attitude, and environment on the quality of life.

The macrobiotic philosophical, social, and biological views have direct practical application. The following suggestions for reducing the day-to-day stresses we all encounter are called "general lifestyle suggestions" and "daily reflections." The first group has to do with our habits in eating, personal hygiene, and living; the second, with our thoughts and attitudes about life.

GENERAL LIFESTYLE SUGGESTIONS

The suggestions that follow aren't hard and fast rules, but neither are they intended to be taken lightly. For as scientists learn more about many of our modern inventions and conveniences such as microwave ovens, television, and chemical-laden "body care" products, more warnings are being placed on more packages, and it is up to the educated and aware consumer to avoid the dangers. Beginning with eating patterns, I will offer some alternatives to several questionable and quite possibly detrimental habits that many of us have fallen into.

Do you drink only when you're thirsty and eat only when hungry? Probably not. Most of us eat and drink too often and too much. The result is fatigue and a widespread problem of obesity.

How do you know when you're hungry? It is basically a question of sensitivity. By eating macrobiotically, you'll find that two to three well-balanced meals, including soup, and two or three cups of tea daily, satisfy hunger and thirst. Of course your needs will depend on your level of activity and the other factors mentioned in Chapter 1. As long as the meals are properly balanced, you may eat as much as you want (short of stuffing yourself full at each meal). If several hours elapse between meals, you may want to have a snack as well.

Regardless of how much you eat, make sure to chew each bite of food thoroughly. By chewing each bite of food until liquefied, you mix it with digestive enzymes, which are especially important for the proper digestion of complex carbohydrates—the major nutrients in the macrobiotic diet.

Another general suggestion on the matter of eating is to stop late-night snacking. Eating less than an hour or so before bed is unhealthful for two reasons: first, you can't sleep soundly while your belly is full of food; and second, you can't digest food properly while your body is half asleep. The result is stagnation in the intestines and a less than adequate night's rest.

In addition to changing eating habits, there are other ways in which to reduce day-to-day stress.

One of these ways is to sleep soundly and peacefully. To achieve this, I recommend that you retire before midnight as often as possible and wake up around sunrise. Sleep researchers have determined that we get our most regenerating rest between 9:00 pm and 1:00 am.

For personal hygiene, it is preferable to wash your skin with pure soap, and to minimize the use of chemically produced body care products. Most commercial cosmetics and detergent or deodorant soaps are damaging to the healthy bacteria on the skin. After lathering up with soap, it takes one to four hours and plenty of Vitamin C to replace the so-called "acid mantle." It is best to use small quantities of pure soap under the arms, around the genitals, and on the face, hands and feet—and as shampoo. On the rest of the body, use a hot, damp washcloth or loofah sponge and rub vigorously instead. This will stimulate healthy blood circulation to the skin and better elimination through the pores. Avoid taking lengthy hot baths or showers.

In addition, try replacing commercial cosmetics with the natural products available in natural foods stores. For example, you may want to use sesame or peanut oil as a moisturizer, oatmeal or clay as a facial pack, herb teas for a facial steam, and lemon juice or cider vinegar diluted with water as an astringent.

All fabrics used close to the skin ought to be as natural as possible. Try to gradually shift from nonabsorbent synthetic-fiber clothes to more comfortable and absorbent cotton, linen, silk, or wool clothes.

Around your home try to replace synthetic towels, sheets, blankets, and carpets with natural fiber ones. Incandescent full-spectrum lighting is better than fluorescent lights, and wooden furniture also contributes to a more healthful atmosphere. House plants freshen and oxygenate the air inside your home, contributing to a cheerful, relaxed environment.

Even in the winter it is a good idea occasionally to open windows to permit fresh air to circulate. During colder weather try not to keep your home overly warm. A slightly cool indoor temperature will help your body adapt better to the cold outdoors. In summer, try using a fan rather than air conditioning. Let your internal bodily thermostat take over from the one on the wall.

Planting a vegetable garden in the springtime is a wonderful thing. Learning to grow and harvest your own food is a rewarding experience. The soil is life itself, and spending time building it and nurturing plants as they grow can transfer that life to your body. If you don't have space to grow vegetables, try flowers.

A number of the modern convenience items many of us take for granted, such as hair dryers, electric toothbrushes, and microwave ovens, may not be good for our health. Modern testing instruments and biofeedback have shown that virtually all electrical appliances sap human energy when they are operated close to the body for extended periods of time. Appliances produce positive ions, which carry an electrical charge opposite to the ions created by growing plants, a waterfall, or rain. Negative ions are known to have a calming effect. Exposure to positive ions from fluorescent lighting, or from sitting in front of electric and electronic machines all day long, may be harmful. If your work demands that you expose yourself to positive ionization, that is all the more reason to avoid it at home.

Another item almost everyone takes for granted is the television set. Color sets especially have been known to emit low-level radiation. The best way to protect yourself from potential harm is, of course, by avoiding television. The next best thing is to watch it at a distance of about fifteen feet.

Macrobiotics doesn't favor a return to some past way of life. It appreciates, values, and continues to use some of the technological advances of modern society. However, many home appliances and cooking devices are unnecessary, and artificially and synthetically produced goods may contribute to the development of illness.

DAILY REFLECTIONS

These "daily reflections" are suggestions for ways of thinking in tune with nature and with good health. At first it will be helpful to set aside a few minutes each day to ponder the ideas. In time you will find yourself being reminded of these calming thoughts no matter where you are or what you are doing.

The first idea is simply to appreciate nature. The way you do this is up to you. You may take a walk in the woods, paint a picture of a tree, write a poem, or sit outside on the porch. Whatever you do, try to leave the cares of your day behind. There will be plenty of time to work them out later. Let this brief period be only for you and thoughts of nature.

Changing the way you eat, dress and live tends to keep you focused for a time on the reasons why you are making these changes. While it is important to be focused on your new directions, try to avoid being preoccupied with the state of your health. Keep active physically and mentally.

Try to encourage family members, especially your spouse, to make positive living changes with you. Unfortunately, not everyone receives the support of a spouse, family, or friends in their wish to eat macrobiotically. Understand that those close to you want the best for you, regardless of how it seems. The best way to gain the support of others is to give them yours. Show them that you care about them and they will do the same for you.

Be grateful for all you have, for your grandparents and their parents who made it possible for you and your parents to be here. If you have the inclination, reconstruct your family tree. Find out how far back you can trace your roots. Most libraries have books that can help you do this.

At mealtimes, be thankful for your food and the company you have to share it with. Let the thanks come from a place deep inside you. A moment of silence or a short prayer before meals gives you an opportunity to slow down, while your body prepares itself for the food. It is the best time to let go of all the worries and responsibilities that can interrupt smooth digestion.

Finally, the expression "one grain, ten thousand grains" relates a great truth of nature. For every seed of wheat given to the earth at planting time, the earth eventually returns ten thousand, even ten million, at the harvest. In the same way, share the love and energy you receive to help others achieve better health and happiness. Teaching others is the best way to learn something for yourself. By teaching them about macrobiotics you will fortify it in yourself.

The lifestyle suggestions and daily reflections can help you along the road to self-discovery, self-knowledge, and better health, improving not only the quality of your own life, but increasing the happiness and joy of those around you.

Beating Diabetes

Larry Bogoslaw's Story

I had always liked sweets, and I had a problem with bedwetting since I was four, but I never had any real problems with my health until October, 1972, when I was eight years old. I remember the night of my cousin's bar mitzvah: I hadn't eaten all day, and I was so hungry by the end of the evening that I binged on as much cake as I could eat. The next morning I threw up and began to feel really fatigued. My mother took me to a pediatrician, and the diagnosis was Type I diabetes; I was put on one shot of insulin per day.

I lacked the willpower to stay on the structured diet plan I was given. By the time I was eleven another doctor put me on two shots of insulin a day in an effort to better control my blood sugar, since I wasn't eating as carefully as I was supposed to. From the start, I was always a very undisciplined eater and drinker, and very poor at following any doctor's instructions; in fact, developing the ability to be orderly and disciplined in my approach to taking care of myself has been one of the biggest changes I have experienced now in my year of practicing macrobiotics. I recall always being angry in the first few years. I had cut sugar out of my diet, but I was still eating plenty of meat.

In 1980 my father discovered macrobiotics in Philadelphia through the East West Foundation. Although my father began eating macrobiotically, I didn't begin until I came to Boston in June, 1983, where I had my first macrobiotic consultation and was given a completely different way to eat right away. At this time I was taking 65 units of insulin a day. Marc Cauwenberghe, the consultant I saw, told me I could possibly be taking as little as 5 or 10 units of insulin by the end of the summer, and I was sure he was crazy! After about ten days of eating macrobiotically, I was able to decrease my insulin dosage, dropping by 10 percent increments, from 65 units to 46 units. By June 20th it was down to 35 or 40 units, and some time in July it went down to 30. Early in August, an experienced macrobiotic cook moved into the apartment where my father and I were staying, and after a short period of eating her cooking, my insulin suddenly took another leap downwards.

In addition to the decrease in my insulin intake, I soon noticed a number of other changes. My acne diminished to a few small, dull bumps on my cheeks, and my complexion was brighter; my shoulders were suddenly straighter; and my energy calm and consistent from 8 A.M. to midnight. As the weeks became months these changes were accentuated, and more deep-seated transformations became apparent as well. Most importantly, it became clear that one old, deeply ingrained assumption of mine was no longer true. This was the assumption that I would not live past the age of thirty-five. With the constant feeling of my vitality ebbing away, every year and every month, this was a constant background in my awareness and approach to life. Now my daily insulin dosage is down to about 15 units, my vitality is ever increasing, and I am enjoying every minute of it, since I know that all my dreams, all my potential will be realized. If I can change this much in a year, anybody else can change, too! ■

By John Mann. Reprinted by permission of Larry Bogoslaw and the author.

12

Balancing the
Macrobiotic Diet

In addition to regular exercise, a more natural lifestyle, and foods high in complex carbohydrates, fiber, vitamins, and minerals, we need a balanced diet. Correct balancing of the macrobiotic diet promotes harmony between the immediate environment and the body, and allows for flexibility in designing a diet that best suits personal nutritional requirements.

As we discussed in Chapter 1, eating locally grown foods is fundamental to the macrobiotic way. Locally grown foods help the body to adapt to seasonal changes, thus preventing seasonal imbalances such as colds or flu, as well as more serious illnesses. There are other important advantages to eating local foods, not the least of which is a cooler body in the heat and a warmer one in the cold.

The human body expands in heat and contracts in cold. A warm water bath, for example, soothes and relaxes (expands) tight muscles, whereas a cold bath stimulates and invigorates (contracts) them. During summer a wrist watch fits more tightly as a result of expansion of the body, while in winter it fits more loosely. The summer season, which is yang, creates a more yin (expanded) body condition. Winter creates the reverse. The food we eat affects the expansion and contraction of the body as well.

During summer we tend to eat more yin foods, and use lighter cooking for balance. We emphasize foods rich in Vitamin C, especially garden vegetables, along with summer grains such as corn, which have an expansive effect on the body and keep us cool. After the autumn harvest, the transition to the yin season (winter) begins. With it the body becomes more yang (contracted). To encourage the change we eat more yang vegetables such as winter squashes, root vegetables, cabbage, and hardy greens, and autumn grains such as oats, wheat, and buckwheat. We also increase the amount of fats and protein foods such as beans and white-meat fish. These foods, coupled with longer cooking times, keep the body warmer and more comfortable during winter.

While it is best to select fresh foods from your immediate locality, you may use other foods brought in from greater distances. In general, more perishable items are best when harvested locally; more readily storable foods, such as grains, beans, sea vegetables, and sea salt need not be of local origin. The table below provides some guidelines for determining the ideal geographic ranges for foods and ingredients imported to your area.

Table 12.1 Geographic Ranges

Food or Ingredient	Ideal Geographic Range
Water	Immediate environment; ideally from a well or clear spring near your home.
Fruit	Same climatic and geographical region; for example, the New England area for someone in Massachusetts, or the southern states for someone in Alabama.
Vegetables	More extended area, but similar to the place in which you live; for example, the New England, mid-Atlantic and mid-western states for someone in New England.
Whole Grains and Beans	Further extended areas that share similar geographical and climatic conditions; for example, anywhere in North America for people living in the United States.
Sea Vegetables	Even further extended than the above; generally anywhere within the same climatic belt; for example, people living in North America or Europe may eat sea vegetables from either place or from temperate zones of the Far East.
Sea Salt	The entire hemisphere, either Northern or Southern, depending upon where you live.

THE ADAPTABILITY OF THE MACROBIOTIC DIET

Within the continental United States, there are differences in climate and environment which you may consider when adapting the macrobiotic diet, and especially cooking styles, to your individual needs.

Table 12.2   Modifications for Climatic Factors

	Lower	Higher
Temperature	More thorough cooking; stronger seasoning	Shorter cooking times; less seasoning
Humidity	More water in cooking	Less water in cooking

In the southern portions of the United States, where temperatures can soar over one hundred degrees for days at a time during the summer, lighter eating is appropriate. As previously mentioned, a diet of whole grains, lightly cooked summer garden vegetables, light soups, pressed and raw salads, and some fruit, keeps the body cool and comfortable.

In more northerly or mountainous regions where the climate is cooler, and during winter, the macrobiotic diet consists of a greater proportion of hearty foods—beans, seeds, nuts, oils, soyfoods, and fish. Longer cooking times are used to generate more body warmth. In macrobiotic cooking for cooler regions, local apples, pears, or dried fruits stewed or baked into desserts replace the fruits or juices used in warmer areas.

BALANCING YIN AND YANG IN THE DIET

Understanding the subtle balancing of foods in the macrobiotic diet in terms of yin and yang is important for personal adaptations of the diet. In general, the modern diet is comprised of extreme foods which can cause the body to become simultaneously too yin and too yang. The typical modern diet tends to foster an expanded (or yin) outer appearance of the body, together with inner rigidity and hardness (an overly yang internal state). The most obvious outward sign of this is overweight. Internally, the extreme yang condition is manifested as tense, tight muscles, stiffness in the joints, accumulation of excess fats and water, and hardening of the arteries.

Eating macrobiotically leads to a more yang appearance; the body becomes slimmer, with better muscle definition and more graceful contours. Internally, the body becomes more balanced, functioning more smoothly and efficiently. The overall benefits of this more balanced condition include increased flexibility and capacity for relaxation.

However, if fish and overcooked, excessively salty, relatively yang foods are over-emphasized in the diet, the individual may experience strong cravings for yin foods such as ice cream, sugared desserts, or alcoholic beverages. When macrobiotic meals are balanced in terms of yin and yang, cravings for extreme foods are minimized, and the body becomes more fit and flexible gradually, at a natural pace.

Whole grains, which are a major component of the macrobiotic diet, are centrally balanced. That is, they are neither too yin nor too yang. However, since different cooking methods affect the subtle balancing of yin and yang, even in whole grains, it is important to understand the qualities of all the foods on the macrobiotic diet, and to select a wide variety of them in your daily meals.

Beans, which are more yin because of their higher protein and fat content, are balanced when cooked with a relatively yang sea vegetable, such as kombu. Vegetables (more yin) are balanced by a little tamari soy sauce or sea salt (more yang). Fruits are also more balanced in terms of yin and yang when they are cooked with a pinch of sea salt.

An afternoon or evening meal that includes miso soup, which, because of its salty taste and high mineral content, is relatively yang, is balanced by the addition of fresh lightly steamed vegetables, a pressed salad or pickled vegetables, and bancha tea (all more yin). A breakfast consisting of miso soup, whole oats, or another whole grain cereal is balanced by garnishes such as chopped scallions, chopped chives, or toasted nori. Cooked fruit, apple butter, or a few raisins may be used occasionally to balance a breakfast meal.

Fish or seafood (yang) is balanced by the addition of vegetables, such as leafy greens and grated raw daikon, or by garnishes or seasonings such as scallion, ginger, or natural mustard (all more yin). Soba noodles, which are more yang, are balanced by the addition of chopped scallions or a liquid broth.

Desserts made from fresh fruit and whole grains or whole grain flour are more yin. When used occasionally, they help satisfy the natural desire for sweets, while the body becomes more healthy. Ending meals with a small amount of naturally sweet foods such as plain brown rice or bancha tea reduces the craving for desserts. When meals reflect the proper balance of yin and yang, they are flavorful, satisfying, and visually appealing.

HOW TO USE THE MACROBIOTIC DIET

Changing the eating habits of a lifetime is quite a challenge, but one well worth the effort. Unless you are in poor health and are being counseled on a regular basis by a qualified macrobiotic counselor, a gradual, yet steady, transition to the macrobiotic diet is best.

Begin by reducing the amount of saturated fats, refined starches, and sugars in your diet. Eat whole grains, vegetables, beans, and sea vegetables more frequently. Always try to avoid foods that are high in cholesterol, saturated fats, sugar, and additives. Use the transitional foods listed in Appendix D as replacements for any of the foods you miss.

An essentially vegetarian macrobiotic diet, with the limited use of animal products, fish, and sweeteners, may be of benefit during recovery from certain serious illnesses. In addition, there are many traditional and natural home remedies that can be used as a part of home health care. The external application of compresses and plasters, and special combinations of foods and condiments, may be extremely helpful in certain cases. Appendix B has information about a few of the more common preparations. Because each person and situation is unique, however, the best way to become acquainted with these home remedies is to visit a macrobiotic information center for guidance from an experienced macrobiotic counselor.

EATING MACROBIOTICALLY

It is best to eat a large variety of wholesome foods, but it isn't necessary, or even healthful, to eat them all at the same meal. An average macrobiotic meal might consist of a bowl of soup, a dish made from one or two whole grains, a few different cooked vegetables, a bean dish or a small serving of white-meat fish, and perhaps a small salad. Eating macrobiotically means understanding the importance of balance, in both the selection and preparation of foods.

When cooking, use a variety of seasonings, rather than always relying on tamari or sea salt alone for flavor. Also use a variety of cooking styles, such as nishime, sautéing, pressure cooking, boiling, baking, and steaming.

Maintaining the ideal proportions of whole grains, vegetables, beans, and the supplementary foods is important (see Figure 1.2). Keep in mind, however, that not every meal need be balanced just so; it is more important to balance the foods eaten during the course of the day. For example, if breakfast consists of miso soup, oatmeal, toast with apple butter, and bancha tea (essentially a whole-grain meal), then the lunch and dinner meals ought to include more vegetables and supplementary foods in relation to whole grains. However, it is important to include whole grains at every meal.

Every day, try to use two or three different whole grains; seven or more different vegetables of varied colors, some eaten raw (pickled or pressed), and some cooked; a sea vegetable or two; and at least one kind of bean or soyfood. If you are healthy you may use white-meat fish a few times per week.

Eat at least two and preferably three meals a day. If you get hungry between meals, have a snack such as a rice cake. Eat enough food to maintain your ideal weight. To lose weight while eating macrobiotically, you needn't count calories; merely follow the standard macrobiotic diet, and eat few, if any, snacks and desserts. To gain weight, do the reverse. Once your weight has stabilized, eat the widest possible variety of recommended foods, while still keeping meals simple.

From Pill-Popping to Pain-Free

Elaine Nussbaum's Story

In April 1980, I had a diagnostic procedure done to determine the cause of the excessive and prolonged menstrual bleeding I was experiencing. The doctor discovered a malignant tumor—a carcinosarcoma in the connective tissue on the wall of the uterus. I was given twenty radiation treatments, a radium implant, hormone medication, and both oral and intravenous chemotherapy. In August, 1980 the doctor performed a radical hysterectomy and a "bilateral salpingo oophorectomy"—the removal of my ovaries. I continued to take chemotherapy.

In May, 1982 I started having pain in the lower back, and despite medication, it got progressively worse. I could neither sit nor lie down. In August, after a few days of standing up day and night, sleeping only on my husband's shoulder in a standing position, I went to an orthopedist. He confirmed a compression fracture and noted also that my vertebrae were partially collapsed. In order to prevent a total collapse of the vertebrae, I was put into a brace which extended from above the chest to the pelvic area and around the back.

The pain got worse and spread to my legs. I could no longer stand. My husband put me in a reclining chair and gave me strong pain-killers around the clock. Nothing stopped the pain.

In September I was carried to the hospital for more X-rays and scans. In addition to the compression fracture and the partially collapsed vertebrae, these pictures showed cancer on the lumbar spine, cancer on the thoracic spine, and multiple metastatic deposits on both lungs.

I was given radiation again (a series of five treatments), then chemotherapy, then five more radiation treatments, then more chemotherapy. The usual program was ten rounds of chemotherapy, given at three to four week intervals. I was tired, weak, nauseous, and in pain.

In January 1983, after four cycles of chemotherapy, X-rays and scans were taken again. The tests showed that there was increased activity and progression of the cancer in the spine, and unchanged metastatic cancer in both lungs.

Towards the end of January, while opening the mail, I cut my finger on an envelope. Because my blood levels were so depressed from the chemotherapy, I was unable to fight the infection that set in. The paper-cut resulted in a ten-day hospital stay, including four blood transfusions, massive doses of intravenous antibiotics, and three days in isolation. It was decided that the chemotherapy I was getting was too strong; I would be put on something less toxic.

It was then I knew that conventional medicine was not going to work for me. I did some research on alternative methods, and I chose macrobiotics. Dr. Sattilaro's book, *Recalled by Life,* was a great inspiration to me. I felt that if he could get well on such a program, I could too. In mid-February I started to wean myself away from meat, dairy products, fruit, and sugar, and to reduce to zero the thirty-eight pills I was taking daily. By the end of February, I was on a macrobiotic diet.

I began the diet in a hospital bed, a wheelchair, and a brace. In a short while, I started walking with a walker, then with a cane. In April, a urinary problem that had plagued me for three years (a result of the original radiation) disappeared. In mid-May I took off the brace. On May 22, I walked up and down my block all by myself.

In June, I put away my wig; my hair, which had all fallen out from the chemotherapy, had grown back enough to be presentable. I returned the hospital bed. I started driving again. I resumed my studies towards my master's degree. In six months, I changed from a sick, depressed, pill-popping invalid to a happy, optimistic, and very grateful pain-free person.

The side effects of the diet have been mostly positive. I have had a few bouts with diarrhea, fatigue, flaky skin, and other non-debilitating forms of "discharge." On the positive side, I enjoy good health, good energy, and perfect bodily functions, such as appetite, sleep, elimination, and mental alertness. And I really enjoy the food—my whole family does too.

Although I take no treatments or medications, I continue to see my oncologist periodically for check-ups. She says that I am doing very well.

I have been practicing macrobiotics now for almost two years. I have completed a masters of science degree in nutrition. My thesis was entitled "Macrobiotics—an Alternative Treatment for Cancer." I am doing nutritional consulting and helping many people with all kinds of degenerative diseases and other illnesses to improve their health. In addition, I teach macrobiotic cooking classes and lecture throughout the New York–New Jersey area.

I attribute the reversal of my cancer solely to macrobiotics, and I hope that my story will be a source of hope and inspiration to others. ■

13

The Macrobiotic Kitchen

Your success with the macrobiotic diet begins in the kitchen. Preparing nutritionally balanced and tasty macrobiotic food is an exciting endeavor, especially if you plan to involve your spouse or other family members in this new way of eating. This chapter will describe kitchen equipment and how it is used, basic cooking techniques, and menu planning. These suggestions will not only save you time and energy, but may mean the difference between mediocre and optimal results.

KITCHEN EQUIPMENT

To begin cooking macrobiotic meals you may need to make an investment in a few kitchen items. You might have them already, but if not, don't try to do without them. By and large, these items are not costly, and they will pay for themselves in countless ways. A stainless steel pressure cooker is the first piece of equipment you will need (see Figure 13.1). It is used often in the macrobiotic kitchen to prepare grains and sometimes beans. The 4-quart size is recommended. In addition, an assortment of stainless steel and cast iron cooking pots is necessary for cooking soups, vegetables, beans, and grains. Such an assortment might include four stainless steel saucepans (two 3-quart, one 2-quart, one 1-quart), a 6-quart cast iron Dutch oven, a cast iron skillet 9 inches in diameter, and one oven-proof baking dish (3-quart size). For baking, heat-resistant glass or earthenware casseroles, bread pans, and pie plates are best.

Figure 13.1   Pressure Cooker

You may be accustomed to using aluminum pots and pans, or cookware coated with a non-stick finish. If you use aluminum cookware often, your blood and bones may absorb aluminum, possibly leading to a toxic condition. Metabolic dysfunctions associated with aluminum poisoning include anemia, headaches, liver and kidney problems, and colitis.

The plastic non-stick coating in pots and pans is easily scratched, and often flakes off and gets cooked in with food. As the stability of this plastic material once it reaches the digestive tract is questionable, and its long-term effects on human health are unknown, it is best to avoid non-stick as well as aluminum cookware.

Metal cooking utensils, especially knives and spoons, are sometimes coated with aluminum, cadmium, lead, or chemical agents during manufacture. Wooden utensils are therefore recommended. Obtain a few inexpensive utensils such as large wooden spoons or ladles, bamboo rice paddles, a roasting paddle, and chopsticks (see Figure 13.2). Stainless steel flatware is appropriate for general table use, while ceramic spoons are especially good for eating soups.

It is best to minimize the use of electric devices in your kitchen. Foods cooked on electric ranges require heavier seasoning, particularly more salt, because they tend to be more bland than gas-cooked foods. There is also an increased possibility that foods cooked by electricity will be burnt, since it is difficult to control the temperature on electric ranges.

Microwave ovens, in which electromagnetic radiation is used to generate heat, damage the foods cooked in them and can harm the user's health as well. Over a period of years, the consumption of foods cooked on electric ranges or in microwave ovens tends to

Figure 13.2   Some Recommended Cooking Utensils

draw the body out of balance, and may lead to severe health problems. If you replace your electric stove with a gas one, you will notice a difference in your food immediately, and your health will improve as well.

Flat metal flame deflectors with wooden handles (see Figure 13.3) are recommended for use when you cook with gas. The flame deflector, which is placed under a pot or pressure cooker during slow cooking of grains, helps to distribute the flame more evenly and prevent burning. Metal deflectors are preferable to ones made of asbestos, a known carcinogen.

Figure 13.3   Flame Deflector

For preparing vegetables, a natural-bristle vegetable scrub brush and a good sharp vegetable knife are indispensable. A Chinese or Japanese style knife made of carbon or stainless steel is especially handy for cutting and chopping. In addition, you will need a sharpening stone and some good-quality wooden cutting boards. It is best to use one fairly large board for cutting vegetables and another, smaller one for fish, because wooden boards are somewhat porous and it is difficult to completely remove the fish odors.

To store seeds, grains, beans, and other dried goods, gallon-sized storage containers with covers are excellent. Glass jars and ceramic or wooden containers are best, because unlike plastic or metal, they do not affect the smell or taste of the foods stored in them. Several smaller glass containers with covers for storing teas, condiments, and spices will also be helpful. One more container that you will use often in cooking is a tamari soy sauce dispenser (see Figure 13.4).

For washing dried beans, sea vegetables, grains, and seeds before soaking or cooking, you will need a large wire mesh strainer (2- or 3-quart size). This can double as a colander for washing vegetables or draining noodles. A smaller fine mesh strainer is good for washing items such as sesame seeds and millet. It can also be used to strain tea, although a small, inexpensive bamboo tea strainer (see Figure 13.4), used only for teas, is ideal. The teas themselves can be brewed in a covered pot or pan—or, of course, in a glass or ceramic teapot.

Tamari Soy Sauce Dispenser

Bamboo Tea Strainer

Figure 13.4

Grater

Suribachi and Surikogi

Figure 13.5

For grating vegetables and ginger root, a hand-held grater that permits fine grating is especially helpful (see Figure 13.5). A stainless steel food mill is convenient for puréeing baby foods and soups. A grinding bowl such as a Japanese suribachi (see Figure 13.5), with a wooden pestle, is necessary for making sesame salt and other condiments, sauces, and dressings. A 6-inch suribachi is good for regular use.

A steamer basket, a pickle press, and a few inexpensive bamboo mats are the other kitchen items that are used most regularly in the preparation of macrobiotic meals. A steamer basket, preferably one made of stainless steel or bamboo, is essential for cooking vegetables and reheating cooked grains (see Figure 13.6). A pickle press (see Figure 13.7) is useful for preparing pressed salads and

stainless steel steamer

bamboo steamer

Figure 13.6   Steamers

Pickle Press   **Bamboo Sushi Mat**

Figure 13.7

pickles; however, you may also make these in a heavy crock, by simply covering the vegetables with a wooden or ceramic plate that fits inside the crock, and setting a weight on top. Bamboo mats (see Figure 13.7) will serve you well, especially in the preparation of sushi, a dish made of rice and vegetables or fish rolled in sheets of toasted nori sea vegetable.

Of course, you are not limited to using only these kitchen items. But if you use others, make sure they are made of wood, cast iron, stainless steel, glass, or earthenware. If you own a stainless steel wok, it will come in handy for sautéing vegetables and noodles; if not, you may use a stainless steel or cast iron skillet to serve the same purpose. Electrical appliances such as blenders, popcorn makers, waffle irons, blenders, and juicers are rarely used to make macrobiotic meals.

STOCKING YOUR SHELVES

If you choose to follow the macrobiotic diet you will be embarking on a whole new way of life. Eventually you may want to clean out your shelves and cupboards, replacing processed and refined items with whole foods. Almost all of these can be found in a good natural foods store; if they are not available in your area, they can be ordered by mail. The table below lists the foods and condiments that you may wish to include in your kitchen. If you wish to adopt the macrobiotic way of life more gradually, you may wish to refer to Appendix D for suggestions about replacing conventional recipe ingredients with more healthful alternatives.

Table 13.1   Things to Have on Hand

SHELVES AND CUPBOARDS

Beans	Aduki, black beans, black soybeans, chick peas, kidney beans, lentils, Lima beans, pinto beans, soybeans, split peas, whole dried peas.
Beverages	Apple juice, bancha tea, grain coffee, mu tea, roasted barley tea, spring water.
Condiments and Seasonings	Barley malt, brown rice vinegar, gomashio, kelp-sesame salt, miso, nori condiment, raisins and other dried fruits, roasted sea vegetable powders, tamari soy sauce, tekka, umeboshi plums, yinnie (rice) syrup.
Dried Fruits	Apples, apricots, cherries, currants, peaches, pears, prunes, raisins.
Dried or Powdered Vegetables	Daikon, ginger, onions, parsley, shiitake mushrooms.
Flour and Flour Products	Buckwheat, cornmeal, rye, sourdough bread, tortillas, unyeasted bread, unleavened crackers, whole wheat (regular and pastry).
Grains	Barley, bulghur wheat, corn, couscous, kasha (roasted buckwheat groats), millet, rice cakes, rolled oats, short and medium grain brown rice, sweet brown rice, wheatberries, whole oats, whole rye.
Noodles	Ramen (whole wheat, rice, buckwheat), soba (buckwheat), somen (fine whole wheat), udon (whole wheat), other whole wheat pastas.
Sea Vegetables	Agar-agar, arame, dulse, hijiki, Irish moss, kelp, kombu, nori, wakame, powdered sea vegetables.
Seeds and Nuts	Pumpkin, sesame, sunflower; almonds, chestnuts, pecans, roasted peanuts, walnuts.

Table 13.1—*Continued*

REFRIGERATOR

Fish and Seafoods	A changing variety, including carp, clams, cod, flounder, haddock, halibut, herring, oysters, scallops, scrod, shrimp, smelts, sole, trout, and other salt and freshwater white-meat fish.
Fruits	A seasonal variety, including apples, apricots, blackberries, blueberries, cantaloupe, cherries, grapes, honeydew melon, peaches, pears, plums, raspberries, strawberries, and watermelon.
Oils	Unrefined corn, safflower, sesame (dark and light); peanut butter, sesame butter, or tahini.
Sweeteners	Apple juice or cider, barley malt, fresh fruit, rice malt or yinnie (rice) syrup.
Vegetables	Broccoli, Brussels sprouts, burdock, cabbages, carrots, cauliflower, daikon, daikon greens, kale, leeks, lettuce, lotus root, mushrooms, mustard greens, parsley, parsnips, pumpkins, radishes, rutabagas, scallions, snow peas, squashes, turnip greens, watercress.
Miscellaneous	Amasake, dried tofu, fu, ginger, horseradish, mochi, natto, natural mustard, peas, pickled vegetables, popping corn, sauerkraut, seitan, tempeh, tofu.

AT HOME IN YOUR KITCHEN

In macrobiotics, proper preparation and cooking of food is as important as the food itself. Proper cooking takes into consideration the ever-changing balance of nature: the various seasons and locations in which individual foods grow; their unique flavors, textures, and energetic qualities; and their relationship to the other foods with which they are cooked and eaten. Proper cooking enhances the flavor of foods, stimulates the appetite, and brings the body into balance. Through subtle changes in food variety, cooking techniques, and seasonings, the macrobiotic cook can continually build health and vitality, while maintaining his or her overall physical and mental balance.

With your kitchen equipment ready and your shelves and refrigerator stocked, you are all set to practice the techniques of macrobiotic food preparation. The ways in which foods are washed, soaked, cut, cooked, and served are all important.

Washing and Soaking

It is important that vegetables be thoroughly washed before they are cut and cooked. It is best not to wash them, however, until you are ready to use them, as they lose their freshness more quickly after they have been washed.

To wash root or ground vegetables, use a natural-bristle vegetable scrubber to remove all soil and dust. Scrub firmly in cold water, being careful not to remove the skin, especially of root vegetables, as it is very nutritious.

It is best to submerge leafy greens in cold water for several seconds before washing them quickly but thoroughly (also with cold water) to remove any sand or soil. Discard any damaged or discolored leaves before washing.

Rinse the sea vegetables wakame, hijiki, arame, and dulse with cold water two or three times. (Instead of rinsing kombu, wipe it with a clean damp cloth.) In most cases, it is also appropriate to soak sea vegetables in cold water for several minutes. Soaking sea vegetables lowers their sodium content, rinses away any dust, and softens them so that they may be sliced easily. Do not soak arame, however, as it will lose much of its flavor and nutritional value.

Before washing grains, place them in a shallow dish or pie plate and remove any stones, sticks, and discolored or damaged grains. To wash, place grains in a large bowl, cover them with cold water, quickly hand-agitate them, and then pour off the water. Repeat this procedure two or three times, until the water is fairly clear. Then pour the grains into a strainer and give them a final quick rinse under cold water to remove any remaining dust and dirt particles. Beans also may be washed in this manner.

Most beans are best soaked for six to eight hours before they are cooked, but it is not necessary to soak lentils and split peas, as they cook very quickly. Soaking is generally recommended because it softens the beans, makes them more digestible, and shortens cooking times. For the same reasons, it may sometimes be appropriate to soak grains such as whole barley, rye, oats, wheat, and (very occasionally) brown rice for six to eight hours.

To soak beans or grains, wash them, place them in a bowl, cover them with water, and set them aside for six to eight hours. Discard the water from soaking beans; the water from soaking grains can be used in cooking to provide additional flavor and nutritive value.

Cutting

Cutting vegetables into various shapes before cooking speeds cooking time (which conserves energy), makes them manageable for eating, and improves texture and appearance. Two other important reasons for cutting vegetables into different shapes are seasonal differences and variety. For instance, if you stir-fry vegetables for a light summer noodle and vegetable dish, you can reduce the amount of time you need to spend in the kitchen by cutting them very thin so that they cook quickly. As for variety, there is no doubt that cutting vegetables into creative shapes adds to their sensory appeal and stimulates the appetite for wholesome fare.

COOKING TECHNIQUES

Macrobiotic cooking differs significantly from several popular cooking styles. In America and parts of Europe, for example, the main ingredient of a meal—usually meat, poultry, or fish—is generally prepared in large pieces, highly seasoned, and served with one or two cooked vegetables, or perhaps with potatoes and a raw salad.

In contrast, the main ingredient of a macrobiotic meal—whole grains—is surrounded by several appealing side dishes made from whole natural ingredients, creating a harmonious combination of flavors, colors, and textures.

Macrobiotic cooking may require more detailed instructions and keener attention to the actual cooking process than you may be accustomed to giving. The simple mixtures and proper cooking methods are important because they take the place of overpowering seasonings and spices in flavoring food. The cooking techniques that are used most regularly in macrobiotic cooking are pressure cooking, boiling, steaming, nishime (waterless cooking), water sautéing, pickling, and pressing. Methods that are used less frequently are oil sautéing, stir-frying, deep frying, baking, and broiling. Raw foods are also used occasionally.

Cooking Whole Grains

To pressure cook whole grains, wash them and place them in the pressure cooker along with the amount of water specified in the recipe. Add a pinch of sea salt, close the cooker, and bring up to pressure. Reduce the flame to medium-low and place a metal flame deflector underneath the cooker to keep the grains from burning. Allow to cook for the amount of time specified in the recipe. For basic information about the operation and maintenance of your pressure cooker, read the manufacturer's instructions.

To boil whole grains, wash them and put them in a pot. Add the amount of cold water specified in the recipe and a pinch of sea salt. Cover the pot, bring to a boil, and then reduce the flame to low. Place a metal flame deflector underneath the pot to prevent burning. Let the grains cook, undisturbed, for the amount of time specified in the recipe. It is best not to stir whole grains while they are cooking.

After grains are cooked, remove them from the heat and allow them to sit undisturbed in the pot or pressure cooker for four to five minutes. You may wish to cook extra grains to be reheated for lunch the next day. Leftover grains can be stored in the refrigerator for several days.

Steaming is not suggested as a way of cooking whole grains, but it is a good method for reheating leftovers. If you use a stainless steel steamer basket, simply place the steamer in about half an inch of water in the pot. Add cooked grain, cover the pot, and bring to a boil. Reduce the flame to low and steam for five minutes or so, until the grain is hot. If you use a bamboo steamer, the same method applies, but you may wish to place the grains on a dinner plate or sauce inside the steamer to prevent them from falling through. If grains are steamed too long, they will get somewhat soggy.

Preparing Quick-Cooking Grains and Whole-Grain Noodles

Precooked grains such as couscous or bulghur wheat are simple to prepare, and they cook quickly. Prepare bulghur wheat by adding it to the amount of boiling water specified in the recipe. Add a pinch of sea salt, cover the pot, and reduce the flame to low. Cook for five to ten minutes, then turn the flame off and let the wheat sit, undisturbed, for about twenty minutes. Remove and fluff up with a spoon. Couscous may be made in the same manner, but the cooking time is less.

The best way to cook whole-grain noodles is quickly, over moderately high heat. Be sure to use plenty of water in a large pot to prevent the noodles from sticking to one another. Bring the water to a boil, add noodles, and cook them, uncovered, until they are tender. Break a noodle apart and check the center to see if it is cooked through. Drain cooked noodles and rinse immediately with cold water.

Cooking Beans

Most beans take longer to cook than whole grains. To prepare the smaller beans, such as split peas and lentils, wash them and add them to the amount of cold water specified in the recipe. Cover the pot, bring them to a boil, and reduce the flame to low. Checking occasionally to make sure that the beans have enough water, cook them for the specified amount of time. Uncover the pot, add sea salt, and continue to cook (uncovered) over low flame, until excess water is boiled off.

Beans such as aduki beans, kidney beans, pinto beans, chick peas, or soybeans are best when they are washed and soaked overnight prior to cooking. To prepare, pour off the water from soaking the beans and place them in a pot. Add the amount of cold water specified in the recipe, along with a strip of kombu sea vegetable. Cover the pot, turn flame to low, and cook for the specified amount of time, checking occasionally to make sure that the beans have enough water. Uncover the pot, add seasoning such as sea salt, miso, or tamari, and continue to cook over low flame until excess water is boiled off.

Beans take less time when cooked in a pressure cooker. With the exception of split peas, lentils, and black soybeans, all types of beans can generally be pressure-cooked. Place soaked beans, kombu, and water in the pressure cooker, cover, and bring up to pressure. Reduce flame to low and cook for the amount of time specified in the recipe. Remove pressure cooker from heat and allow the pressure to drop before adding seasoning such as sea salt, miso, or tamari. Boil off excess water over low flame before serving the beans.

Beans are best when cooked until very soft. Undercooked, starchy-tasting beans are hard to digest. Soaking the beans overnight before cooking helps to soften them, and removes gas-producing compounds. Cooking the beans with kombu also makes them easier to digest. Leftover beans can be added to soups or fried grains, or reheated in a pan with a little water.

Cooking Vegetables

There are many ways to prepare appealing vegetable dishes, including boiling, steaming, sautéing, nishime (waterless cooking), baking, and tempura (deep frying).

To boil vegetables, simply place one-half to one inch of water in a pot, bring water to a boil, and add vegetables. Cook until the vegetables are moist and tender, then remove them and spread them out in a bowl to cool slightly before serving.

To steam vegetables, wash, cut, and then place them in a steamer basket. You may use either a collapsible stainless steel steamer that sets down into a pot, or a bamboo steamer that rests on top. Place about one-half to one inch of water in the pot and bring the water to a boil. Cover steamer and steam vegetables over medium flame until they become tender.

When using a stainless steel steamer, make certain that the steamer basket is above the level of the water. Bamboo steamers have separate sections so that you may stack the vegetables, placing the heavier and thicker ones in the bottom layer and then adding the lighter, leafy vegetables to the top layer a short time later. Steamed vegetables are often crisper than boiled ones.

You may wish to save the water left over from steaming or boiling vegetables for use in soups and recipes requiring vegetable stock. Pour the water into an open jar, let it cool, cover, and refrigerate. The water will keep several days.

To sauté, lightly brush a cast iron skillet, wok, or stainless steel frying pan with sesame oil. For well-done, tender vegetables, heat the skillet, add the vegetables, and cook them over a moderately low flame. Use a high flame if you want crisper, more quickly cooked sautéed vegetables.

To flavor sautéed vegetables, and also to make the oil easier to digest, you may wish to add a pinch of sea salt at the beginning of cooking or a little tamari soy sauce at the end of cooking. Stir the vegetables occasionally while you are sautéing, and add a little water if necessary to prevent them from sticking.

In most cases, sautéed vegetables are best if they remain crisp, but not raw. In some cases they may be cooked soft. Generally, greens are best sautéed very quickly, while roots require a little more time. Thicker cuts of root vegetables require more cooking time than thinner ones. Stir-fried vegetables are prepared like sautéed vegetables, except that the flame is turned slightly higher, and they are stirred frequently until done. They should remain fairly crisp.

Another important cooking method is the nishime style, which is also known as "waterless cooking." Nishime style is a superb way of cooking vegetables without adding oil or allowing nutrients to escape into boiling or steaming water. This cooking method is often recommended for people with illness.

To prepare nishime, place a couple of strips of soaked and sliced kombu sea vegetable in a pot with a heavy lid. Cut vegetables such as carrots, turnips, daikon, onions, burdock, winter squash, or cabbage into two-inch chunks. Place any combination of these on top of the kombu and add one-half to one inch of water. Add a pinch of sea salt, cover the pot, and place over high flame until the water boils. Reduce flame to low and cook for about twenty-five minutes or until vegetables are tender. Season with a small amount of tamari soy sauce and continue to cook about ten minutes longer or until almost all liquid is gone. Mix the vegetables to coat them with any remaining tamari-seasoned juice, remove, and serve.

Other foods that may be included with vegetables in nishime-style cooking are tempeh, fu, dried or fresh tofu, and (as long as you are not cooking for anybody who has a serious illness) pan-fried or deep-fried tofu.

Baking is an especially appropriate method of cooking winter vegetables such as pumpkin or squash. Wash the squash, cut it in half, and place it with the flat side down on a lightly oiled baking sheet. Bake at 375° F until soft. If you are making an oven casserole or vegetable pie, you may steam the vegetables lightly or boil them briefly before baking them in a covered dish.

HOW TO PLAN MACROBIOTIC MEALS

The aim of macrobiotic cooking is to achieve balance and harmony in the body and with the environment. When high-quality natural ingredients are properly prepared, in a calm, peaceful, and loving manner, the result is balanced food that will foster a healthy, balanced condition.

Your challenge as a macrobiotic cook will be in preparing and serving dishes that complement each other in a lively unity—not merely in terms of flavor, but nutritionally and visually as well. The well-planned and well-prepared meal will be as pleasing to the eye as it is to the palate. So whether you are arranging a complete meal on each plate, or simply placing steamed broccoli in a bowl, try to employ your creative talents. A wide variety of serving dishes and trays will help you to vary the presentation of the food you cook. Of course, it is not necessary (or desirable) to have complicated dishes or arrangements of food every day.

Designing a macrobiotic meal is likely to require a bit more thinking ahead and planning than you are used to. You may find Figure 1.2 and the Sample Menus on pages 138–140 to be helpful guides in planning daily menus.

If you read and follow the recipe directions carefully, your first meal will be as good as the rest. As you become more comfortable in your new kitchen, don't be afraid to improvise, using the macrobiotic ingredients discussed throughout this book. You will soon be preparing meals so delectable that people will think you have been cooking this way all your life.

One of the most important aspects of planning and preparing a macrobiotic meal is timing. In general, whole grains, beans, sea vegetables such as kombu and hijiki, and baked vegetables will take the longest to cook, anywhere from fifty minutes to two and a half hours. Pressure cooking will take less time, but cooking all your food in a pressure cooker to save time isn't a good idea, as a variety of cooking techniques is important to macrobiotic cooking and to your health. Miso soup and boiled, steamed, and sautéed foods take about ten to fifteen minutes to prepare, as do noodles, couscous, tofu, natto, and tempeh. Nishime takes about thirty to forty minutes. As the recipes in Chapter 14 indicate, foods such as pickles, sourdough breads, pressed salads, and sauerkraut may take anywhere from several hours to a few days to ferment.

The following sample menus are intended as a guide for beginners. You can experiment further and create lively and tasty combinations of your own. If you are committed to the macrobiotic way of cooking, you have a lifetime of learning ahead of you, for the possibilities are limitless. Along this line, cooking classes offered by macrobiotic cooks can be invaluable.

Table 13.3 Sample Menus

MENU 1

Breakfast	Lunch	Dinner
Soft Rice Cereal	Millet Croquettes	Lentil Soup
Fried Tofu	Chinese-Style Vegetables	Pressure-Cooked Brown Rice
Steamed Broccoli	Rice Bran Pickles	Kinpura Carrots and Burdock
Bancha Tea	Bancha Tea	Boiled Mustard Greens
		Red Radish Pickles
		Raisin-Nut Cookies
		Grain Coffee

MENU 2

Breakfast	**Lunch**	**Dinner**
Miso Soup	Carrot and Watercress Sushi	French Onion Soup
Whole Oats with Raisins		Pressure-Cooked Brown Rice with Aduki Beans
Broccoli Pickles	Steamed Kale	
Gomashio	Fried Tempeh with Ginger	Boiled Turnip Greens
Bancha Tea		Nishime Vegetables
	Bancha Tea	Quick Cucumber Pickles
		Grain Coffee

MENU 3

Breakfast	**Lunch**	**Dinner**
Crisp Brown Rice Cereal	Udon and Broth	Pressure-Cooked Brown Rice and Barley
Amasake	Boiled Tempeh and Scallions	
Chinese Cabbage Pickles		Watercress Soup
Grain Coffee	Garden Salad	Ginger-Broiled Scallops
	Bancha Tea	Boiled Salad with Tempeh
		Nori Condiment
		Blueberry Couscous Cake
		Bancha Tea

MENU 4

Breakfast	**Lunch**	**Dinner**
Buckwheat Pancakes	Whole Grain and Vegetable Patties	Pressure-Cooked Brown Rice
Applesauce		
Steamed Chinese Cabbage	Grated Daikon	Chick Pea Soup
Onion Pickles	Steamed Kale and Carrots	Hijiki Salad
Bancha Tea	Bancha Tea	Boiled Watercress
		Sautéed Burdock with Sesame Seeds
		Bancha Tea

MENU 5

Breakfast	Lunch	Dinner
Soft Millet and Squash	Fried Rice and Vegetables	Pressure-Cooked Brown Rice and Millet
Toasted Nori Strips	Daikon Pickles	Scrambled Tofu
Sauerkraut	Grain Coffee	Puréed Squash Soup
Bancha Tea		Boiled Broccoli
		Pressed Salad
		Stewed Pears
		Bancha Tea

MENU 6

Breakfast	Lunch	Dinner
Soft Barley	Rice Balls or Triangles	Pressure-Cooked Brown Rice
Miso Soup with Wakame and Daikon	Watercress Sushi	Seitan-Barley Soup
Steamed Collard Greens	Broiled Tofu	Watercress Salad
Bancha Tea	Grain Coffee	Dried Daikon and Kombu
		Cucumber Pickles
		Apple-Raisin Kanten
		Bancha Tea

MENU 7

Breakfast	Lunch	Dinner
Mochi	Fried Udon and Vegetables	Pressure-Cooked Brown Rice and Wheatberries
Grated Daikon	Steamed Kale	Clear Broth
Toasted Nori Strips	Grain Coffee	Aduki Beans with Kombu and Squash
Boiled Chinese Cabbage		Arame with Carrots and Onions
Bancha Tea		Boiled Mustard Greens
		Boiled Red Radishes with Umeboshi-Kuzu Sauce
		Bancha Tea

14

Recipes

The recipes in this chapter will introduce you to the delicious variety of macrobiotic cooking. They are generally appropriate for people in good health living in a temperate, four-season climate. Many of the basic cooking techniques discussed in Chapter 13, including boiling, steaming, pressure cooking, sautéing, and nishime, are used, and a number of cutting and serving styles are suggested.

Whole grains, vegetables, and beans make up 80–90 percent of the macrobiotic diet. Recipes emphasizing these ingredients are presented first in this chapter. They are followed by a number of recipes for soups and supplementary foods. As a whole, these simple, easy-to-prepare recipes have been selected to provide practical guidelines for a balanced and nutritious way of eating.

Once you familiarize yourself with the recipes, you can locate any one of them quickly by using the alphabetical index on page 245. Each recipe will serve three or four people. When you are cooking for more than four people, it will take a little more time to wash, cut, and cook the larger volume of food. Use larger pots, and adjust the recipes as needed. If any food is left over, it can be reheated and served for lunch the following day.

Of course, the recipes in this chapter are only a small sampling of the infinite possibilities that you may explore in the world of macrobiotic cooking. When you become adept at basic cooking styles, techniques, and menu planning, you may wish to consult other sources for additional recipes and information about macrobiotic food preparation. There are a number of excellent macrobiotic cookbooks available, and classes with experienced macrobiotic cooking instructors are most helpful.

GRAINS

Grain Entrees

Pressure-Cooked Brown Rice

---

1 cup brown rice
1¼–1½ cups water
pinch of sea salt

Wash rice and place in pressure cooker. Add water and cook over low flame for 10–15 minutes. Add sea salt and place cover on pressure cooker. Turn flame to high and bring cooker up to pressure. Reduce flame to medium-low, place flame deflector under cooker, and cook for 50 minutes.

Remove cooker from flame and allow pressure to come down. Remove cover and let rice sit in cooker for 4–5 minutes. Place rice in a wooden bowl, garnish, and serve.

---

*Pressure-Cooked Brown Rice
with Aduki Beans*

¼ cup aduki beans
1½–1¾ cups water
1 cup brown rice
pinch of sea salt

Wash aduki beans and place in a saucepan with 1½–1¾ cups of water. Bring to a boil, cover, and reduce flame to medium-low. Simmer for 15–20 minutes. Remove from flame and allow beans to cool. Reserve cooking water.

Wash rice and place in pressure cooker. Add cooled beans and cooking water (make sure there are 1½–1¾ cups left; if necessary, add fresh water to make up the difference).

Cook over low flame for 15–20 minutes. Add sea salt and place cover on pressure cooker. Turn flame to high and bring cooker up to pressure. Reduce flame to medium-low, place flame deflector under cooker, and cook for 50 minutes.

Remove from flame and allow pressure to come down. Remove cover and let rice sit in cooker for 4–5 minutes. Serve rice in a wooden bowl.

Pressure-Cooked Brown Rice and Barley

¾ cup brown rice
¼ cup pearled barley
1½ cups water
pinch of sea salt

Wash rice and barley and place in pressure cooker. Add water. Set aside to soak for 4 or 5 hours. After soaking grains, cook over low flame for 10–15 minutes. Add sea salt and place cover on pressure cooker. Turn flame to high and bring cooker up to pressure. Reduce flame to medium-low, place flame deflector under cooker, and cook for 50 minutes.

Remove cooker from flame and allow pressure to come down. Remove cover and let rice and barley sit in cooker for 4–5 minutes. Place grains in a wooden bowl, and serve.

Pressure-Cooked Brown Rice
and Wheatberries

¼ cup wheatberries
¾ cup brown rice
1½ cups water
pinch of sea salt

Soak wheatberries for 6–8 hours or dry-roast them. Wash rice and proceed as directed for Pressure-Cooked Rice and Barley, above.

Pressure-Cooked Brown Rice and Millet

¾ cup brown rice
¼ cup millet
1½ cups water
pinch of sea salt

Wash rice and millet and place in pressure cooker. Add water and cook over medium-low flame for 10–15 minutes. Add sea salt and place cover on pressure cooker. Turn flame to high and bring cooker up to pressure. Reduce flame to medium-low, place flame deflector under cooker, and cook for 50 minutes.

Remove cooker from flame and allow pressure to come down. Remove cover and let rice and millet sit in cooker for 4–5 minutes. Place grains in a wooden bowl, and serve.

Rice Balls or Triangles

---

2 sheets toasted nori (page 177)
4 cups pressure-cooked or boiled brown rice
2 umeboshi plums, halved

Fold both sheets of toasted nori in half and tear along fold. Then fold each section in half again and tear along fold to make a total of 8 equal-sized pieces. Set aside.

Wet your hands slightly in a dish of water with a pinch of sea salt dissolved in it. Take 1 cup of rice and form it into a ball or triangle by cupping your hands into a "V" shape. Pack rice firmly to form a solid ball or triangle. With your thumb, press a hole into the center of the rice and insert ½ umeboshi plum. Firmly pack rice ball or triangle again to close the hole.

Wet your hands slightly and cover rice ball or triangle with 2 pieces of nori, 1 piece at a time, so that it sticks. You may have to wet your hands occasionally to keep rice and nori from adhering to them, but if you use too much water, the rice balls will lose some of their flavor and spoil relatively quickly.

Continue making rice balls or triangles until all rice is used (4 rice balls or triangles). Place on a platter and serve.

Sesame-Coated Rice
Balls or Triangles

---

4 cups pressure-cooked or boiled brown rice
2 umeboshi plums, halved
½ cup roasted sesame seeds (page 191)

Wet your hands very slightly. Take about 1 cup of rice and form it into a ball or triangle by cupping your hands into a ''V' shape. Pack rice firmly to form a solid ball or triangle. With your thumb, press a hole into the center of the rice and insert ½ umeboshi plum. Firmly pack rice ball or triangle again to close the hole. Roll in roasted sesame seeds to coat evenly.

Repeat this process with remaining ingredients to make 4 rice balls or triangles. Place on a platter and serve.

Cucumber Sushi

---

4 sheets toasted nori (page 177)
8 cups pressure-cooked brown rice
1 cucumber, sliced lengthwise into strips
   ½ inch thick
2 tablespoons shiso leaves

Place a sheet of toasted nori on a bamboo sushi mat. Evenly spread about 2 cups of cooked brown rice over the nori sheet, leaving 1 or 2 inches at the top edge and about ¼ inch at the bottom edge uncovered. Press rice down firmly with a slightly damp bamboo rice paddle.

Place 1 or 2 cucumber strips across the width of the nori sheet, ½–1 inch from the bottom. Next, place 3–4 shiso leaves in a row parallel to the cucumber strips.

Use both hands to roll the sushi mat into a cylinder shape, pressing mat firmly against nori and rice. When nori sheet is completely rolled up, wet the top edge lightly with water and press to seal edges tightly. Before unrolling sushi mat, squeeze gently to remove excess liquid.

Wet a sharp vegetable knife and slice nori roll in half. Wet knife again and slice each half into 4 equal sections (rounds), approximately 1 inch thick. You may need to wet knife slightly before making each cut. Repeat entire process with other sheets of nori.

Arrange sushi on an attractive platter with cut side facing up, showing rice and cucumber, and serve.

Carrot and Watercress Sushi

---

2 carrots, quartered lengthwise
16 watercress sprigs
4 sheets toasted nori (page 177)
8 cups pressure-cooked brown rice
4 tablespoons roasted sesame seeds (page 191)

Place about ½ inch of water in a saucepan and bring to a boil. Drop in carrot strips and simmer until tender. Use a slotted spoon or a pair of cooking chopsticks to remove cooked carrots, leaving the water in the pot. Let carrots drain in a colander. Drop watercress springs into cooking water, and boil for about 45 seconds. Remove, drain, and spread out on a plate to cool.

Place a sheet of toasted nori on a bamboo sushi mat. Evenly spread about 2 cups of cooked brown rice over the nori sheet, leaving 1 or 2 inches at the top edge and about ¼ inch at the bottom edge uncovered. Press rice down firmly with a slightly damp bamboo rice paddle.

Place 2 strips of carrot across the width of the nori sheet, about an inch or so from the bottom. Next, place 4 sprigs of watercress in a row alongside carrot strips. Sprinkle about 1 tablespoon of roasted sesame seeds on top of the vegetables.

Use both hands to roll the sushi mat into a cylinder shape, pressing mat firmly against nori and rice. When nori sheet is completely rolled up, wet the top edge lightly with water and press to seal edges tightly. Before unrolling sushi mat, squeeze gently to remove excess liquid.

Wet a sharp vegetable knife and slice nori roll in half. Wet knife again and slice each half into 4 equal sections (rounds), approximately 1 inch thick. You may need to wet knife slightly before making each cut. Repeat entire process with other sheets of nori.

Arrange sushi on an attractive platter with cut side facing up, showing carrot and watercress, and serve.

Tempeh-Sauerkraut Sushi

---

1 pound tempeh
4 sheets toasted nori (page 177)
8 cups pressure-cooked brown rice
8 tablespoons sauerkraut
tamari

Slice tempeh into strips about 6 inches long by ¼ wide by ½ thick. Place in a pot with enough water to almost cover. Cover pot, bring water to a boil, and reduce flame to medium-low. Simmer for 15–20 minutes. Season with tamari and continue cooking, uncovered, until all liquid is gone.

Place a sheet of toasted nori on a bamboo sushi mat. Evenly spread about 2 cups of cooked brown rice over the nori sheet, leaving 1 or 2 inches at the top edge and about ¼ inch at the bottom edge uncovered. Press rice down firmly with a slightly damp bamboo rice paddle.

Place 1 or 2 strips of tempeh across the width of the nori sheet, about an inch or so from the bottom. Place 2 tablespoons of sauerkraut on top of the tempeh.

Use both hands to roll the sushi mat into a cylinder shape, pressing mat firmly against nori and rice. When nori sheet is completely rolled up, wet the top edge lightly with water and press to seal edges tightly. Before unrolling sushi mat, squeeze gently to remove excess liquid.

Wet a sharp vegetable knife and slice nori roll in half. Wet knife again and slice each half into 4 equal sections (rounds), approximately 1 inch thick. You may need to wet knife slightly before making each cut. Repeat entire process with other sheets of nori.

Arrange sushi on an attractive platter with cut side facing up, and serve.

Mochi

---

1 cup sweet brown rice
1–1¼ cups water
pinch of sea salt

Wash sweet rice and place in pressure cooker. Add water. Set aside to soak for 4–6 hours. After soaking sweet rice, add sea salt and place cover on pressure cooker. Turn flame to high and bring cooker up to pressure. Reduce flame to medium-low, place flame deflector under cooker, and cook for 50 minutes.

Remove cooker from flame and allow pressure to come down. Let sweet rice sit in cooker for 4–5 minutes before placing it in a thick wooden bowl. Pound rice with a heavy wooden pestle until all grains are crushed and rice becomes very sticky. You may need to wet the pestle occasionally, but do not use too much water. Good mochi takes about 1 hour to pound.

After pounding rice, oil or flour a cookie sheet (use rice flour) and spread rice out to dry for 1–2 days. Store dried mochi in refrigerator or in a cool dry place.

To toast mochi after it has dried properly, slice into 2-inch squares and place in skillet. Turn flame to medium-low and cover skillet. Toast until mochi is golden brown; then turn it over and toast other side until golden brown. Remove and serve with grated daikon and a few toasted nori strips. Serve each person 2 or 3 slices of mochi.

Fried Rice and Vegetables

1 cup onions, diced
1 cup cabbage, cut into 1-inch
  chunks
½ cup carrots, cut into
  matchsticks
1–2 tablespoons water
4 cups pressure-cooked brown
  rice
1 tablespoon chopped parsley
dark sesame oil
tamari

Heat a small amount of dark sesame oil in a skillet. Sauté onions over high flame for 3–4 minutes. Reduce flame to medium–low and layer cabbage, carrots, and rice on top. Add 1–2 tablespoons water.

Cover skillet, reduce flame to low, and cook until all vegetables are tender and rice is warm and soft. Just before vegetables are done, season with a little tamari and add chopped parsley. Mix rice with vegetables and continue to cook for another 3–5 minutes.

Udon and Broth

1 package (8 ounces) whole wheat
  udon noodles
1 kombu strip, 3–4 inches long, soaked
4 cups water, including water from soaking
  kombu and shiitake
2 or 3 shiitake mushrooms, soaked, stems
  removed, and sliced
2–3 tablespoons tamari

Place about 10 cups of water in a pot and bring to a boil. Stir in udon and cook until noodles are tender and the same color inside and outside. Remove udon from heat and place in strainer. Rinse under cold water and allow to drain.

Place kombu, shiitake, and 4 cups of water in a saucepan. Bring to a boil. Reduce flame to medium-low, cover, and simmer for 5–10 minutes. Remove kombu and set aside for future use. Season soup stock with tamari, reduce flame to low, and simmer for about 5 minutes.

Place a serving of cooked udon in each individual's bowl and pour about 1 cup of hot broth over udon. Garnish each serving with a teaspoon of sliced scallions, and serve.

Fried Udon and Vegetables

> 1 package (8 ounces) whole wheat
> udon noodles
> 1 medium onion, cut into half-moons
> 1 celery stalk, sliced diagonally
> 1 carrot, cut into matchsticks
> dark sesame oil
> tamari

Cook udon, rinse, and drain as directed in the recipe for Udon and Broth. Heat a small amount of dark sesame oil in a skillet. Add onion and sauté for 2–3 minutes over fairly high flame, stirring to cook evenly and prevent burning. Add celery and carrot and sauté for 3–4 minutes. Place noodles on top of vegetables, and cover skillet. Reduce flame to low and cook until vegetables are tender.

Remove cover and season with a little tamari. Mix and sauté for 3–4 minutes longer. Remove, place in a serving bowl, and serve.

Millet Croquettes

> 4 cups pressure-cooked millet
> 1 medium onion, diced (1 cup)
> sesame oil

In a bowl, mix millet and diced onion thoroughly. Wet your hands slightly with cold water. Take about ½ cup of millet mixture and press firmly into a ball. Make sure that ball is packed firmly, or it will fall apart while frying.

Place 2–3 inches of sesame oil in a pot and turn flame to medium. Do not allow oil to smoke or boil. Test temperature by dropping a small amount of millet into it. If oil is not hot enough, millet will stay at the bottom of the pot. If oil is too hot, millet will sink to the bottom but rise back to the surface immediately. If oil is at just the right temperature, millet will first sink to the bottom and then rise to the surface in a few seconds. When oil is at the right temperature, place 2 or 3 millet balls in pot and deep-fry until golden brown. Remove croquettes and drain.

Continue to form balls and deep-fry them until all millet is used (8 croquettes). Place 2 croquettes in each individual's bowl. Pour the sauce from Chinese-Style Vegetables recipe (page 159) over. Garnish with scallions, if desired, and serve.

Home-Made Seitan

3½ pounds whole wheat flour (from hard
    spring or hard winter wheat)
18–20 cups spring water
1 kombu strip, 12 inches long, soaked
3–5 tablespoons tamari

Place flour in a large bowl and add 8–9 cups of warm water to obtain a consistency like oatmeal or cookie batter. Knead for 3–5 minutes, until flour is mixed thoroughly with water. Cover with 4–5 cups of warm water and allow dough to sit for a minimum of 5–10 minutes. Knead again in soaking water for 1 minute. Pour cloudy water into a jar. (This cloudy water is "seitan starch water," and may be saved for use in other recipes.)

Transfer dough to a large strainer and put the strainer in a large bowl or pot. Pour cold water over the dough and knead in the strainer. Drain off cold water. Pour hot water over the dough and knead again. Alternate between cold and hot water when rinsing and kneading, repeating until bran and gluten are completely separated.

Gluten should form a sticky mass. Separate it into 5 or 6 pieces and form balls. Drop balls into 6 cups of boiling water and boil for 5 minutes, or until balls rise to the surface. Add kombu and tamari and cook for 35-45 minutes. (The liquid in the pot is "seitan-tamari water," and may be saved for use in other recipes.)

Slice or cube seitan as called for in a recipe, or store seitan balls in a glass jar in the refrigerator. When stored in the tamari-water mixture, seitan will keep for 4-5 days. The stronger the concentration of tamari, the longer it will keep. Seitan stored in full-strength tamari will keep for several weeks, but it must be soaked in water for about 30 minutes prior to use, to remove excess salt.

Whole Grain and Vegetable Patties

---

4 cups pressure-cooked or boiled millet
1 cup onions, diced
½ cup carrots, diced
¼ cup celery, diced
½ cup cooked seitan, diced, (page 151)
1 cup water
tamari
whole wheat pastry flour or whole
    wheat flour (optional)
dark sesame oil

In a bowl, mix millet and vegetables thoroughly. Mix in seitan. Add water and a small amount of tamari and mix again. Grain should be moist enough so that you will be able to make patties; if necessary, add a little more water. If grain is too moist, add a little whole wheat pastry flour until you obtain the right consistency.

Take 1 handful of grain and vegetable mixture and shape into a patty. Repeat until all grain is gone.

Heat a moderate amount of sesame oil in a skillet. Place several patties in skillet, cover, and reduce flame to medium-low. Cook until golden brown. Turn patties over and cook until golden brown. Remove and place on a serving platter. Garnish with sprigs of fresh parsley.

Cereals, Pancakes, and Bread

Oatmeal with Raisins
---

2 cups rolled oats
½ cup raisins
3 cups water
pinch of sea salt per cup of oats

Heat a stainless steel skillet. Add dry oats, reduce flame to low, and roast oats slowly until they release a nutty fragrance. Stir constantly to avoid burning oats and to roast them evenly.

Place roasted oats in a pot; add raisins, water, and sea salt. Cover and bring to a boil. Reduce flame to medium-low, place flame deflector under pot, and simmer for 25–30 minutes. This cereal may be topped with yinnie (rice) syrup, barley malt, or amasake, or garnished with roasted seeds or nuts.

Soft Rice Cereal
---

1 cup brown rice
5 cups water
pinch of sea salt or ½ umeboshi plum

Wash rice and place in pressure cooker. Add water and sea salt or umeboshi plum. Place cover on pressure cooker and turn flame to high. Bring cooker up to pressure, place flame deflector underneath, and reduce flame to medium-low. Cook for approximately 50 minutes.

Remove cooker from flame and allow pressure to come down. Remove cover and place cereal in individual bowls. Garnish with a few sliced scallions and toasted nori strips or squares, and serve.

Whole Oats with Raisins

1 cup whole oats
5 cups water
½ cup raisins
pinch of sea salt

Place all ingredients in a pot and bring water to a boil. Cover and reduce flame to very low. Place flame deflector under pot and allow to cook overnight so that cereal becomes very soft and creamy. If you do not want to cook overnight, you may pressure cook this cereal: place all ingredients in pressure cooker and cook for 50–60 minutes over medium-low flame, as you would for Soft Rice Cereal. Garnish with Gomashio (page 183) or dulse flakes.

Crisp Brown Rice Cereal

crisp brown rice cereal
amasake

This prepackaged cereal is available at most natural foods stores. Pour amasake (rice milk) over each individual serving.

Soft Millet and Squash

1 cup millet
1 cup buttercup squash *or* Hokkaido
    pumpkin, cut into 1-inch chunks
5 cups water
pinch of sea salt

Wash millet and place in a dry stainless steel skillet. Turn flame to low and dry-roast millet until it releases a nutty fragrance. Stir constantly to roast evenly and prevent burning. Place all ingredients in pressure cooker. Cover cooker and bring up to pressure. Place flame deflector under cooker and reduce flame to medium-low. Cook for 20 minutes.

Remove cooker from flame and allow pressure to come down. Serve millet garnished with chopped scallions or parsley, if desired.

Soft Barley

---

1 cup barley, soaked 6–8 hours
5 cups water
1 kombu strip, 6 inches long, soaked and cut
    into 1-inch squares
¼ cup chopped scallions
1 sheet toasted nori (page 177), cut into
    1-inch squares
pinch of sea salt
tamari (optional)

Place barley, water, and kombu in pressure cooker. Turn flame to high and bring cooker up to pressure. Place flame deflector under cooker and reduce flame to medium-low. Cook for 50 minutes.

Remove cooker from flame and allow pressure to come down. Place cereal in individual serving dishes and garnish with a few chopped scallions, several squares of toasted nori, and 2 or 3 drops of tamari (if desired). Serve.

Buckwheat Pancakes

---

1 cup buckwheat flour
½ cup whole wheat flour or whole wheat
    pastry flour
$1/_8$ teaspoon sea salt
$1^1/_3$ cups water or apple juice
light sesame oil

Combine dry ingredients. Add water or apple juice to create the desired consistency for pancakes. Mix very well with a spoon or whisk. Let batter sit in a warm place overnight so that it begins to ferment. This will help the pancakes to rise and become lighter.

Lightly oil a skillet or pancake griddle with light sesame oil, and heat. Place a small amount of batter on griddle to form a round cake. Fry over medium flame until little air bubbles start to appear on the uncooked side of the pancake. Turn pancake over and fry until golden brown. If flame is too high, pancakes will burn.

Sourdough Bread

Sourdough Starter

1 cup whole wheat flour
spring water

Add enough water to 1 cup whole wheat flour to make a thick batter. Cover with a damp cloth and allow to ferment for 3–4 days in a warm place.

Bread Dough

8 cups whole wheat flour *or* 5 cups whole
wheat flour and 3 cups rye flour
¼–½ teaspoon sea salt
2 tablespoons sesame oil (optional)
spring water

Mix flour and salt, add oil, and sift thoroughly together by hand.

Sourdough Bread

Mix in 1–1½ cups of sourdough starter when making bread dough. Knead 300–350 times. (For variety, you may knead in 1½–2 cups diced onion, 1½–2 cups raisins, or ½–1 cup roasted seeds or nuts.)

Oil 2 bread pans with sesame oil and dust with flour. Place dough in pans and cover with a damp cloth. Let sit for 8–12 hours in a warm place. After dough has risen, bake at 200° F for ½ hour and then for 1 hour or so at 350° F.

Serve each person 1 or 2 slices of toasted sourdough bread.

VEGETABLE DISHES AND SALADS

Vegetable Entrees

Boiled Mustard Greens

---

4 cups mustard greens
water

Slice mustard greens diagonally. Place about 1 inch of water in a pot and bring to a boil. Add mustard greens, cover, and reduce flame to medium-low. Cook for 2–3 minutes so that the greens are slightly crisp and bright green in color. Remove, drain, and place in a serving bowl. You may toss the greens several times with cooking chopsticks or wooden spoons to cool them slightly so that they retain their bright color.

Mustard greens may also be cooked whole. Cook as described above; remove, drain, and allow to cool slightly. Using both hands, shape greens into a roll or cylinder shape, and squeeze out most of the liquid. Slice roll into 1½–2 inch pieces and arrange attractively on a serving platter.

Boiled Turnip Greens

---

4 cups turnip greens, sliced diagonally into
   2-inch pieces
¼ cup roasted sesame or sunflower seeds
   (page 191)
water

Place about 1 inch of water in a pot and bring to a boil. Add turnip greens, cover, and reduce flame to medium-low. Simmer for 2–3 minutes, until greens are tender but still bright green. Remove, drain, and place in a serving bowl. You may toss the greens several times with wooden spoons or cooking chopsticks to allow them to cool. Sprinkle roasted sesame seeds or sunflower seeds on top for garnish, and serve.

Boiled Watercress

2 bunches of watercress
4 lemon slices, cut into thin half-moons
water

Place about 1 inch of water in a pot and bring to a boil. Place 1 bunch of watercress in the boiling water. Simmer for 45–50 seconds, stirring or mixing to cook evenly. Use a slotted spoon or a pair of cooking chopsticks to remove cooked watercress, leaving the water in the pot. Drain watercress in a colander. Boil the remaining watercress in the same way; remove and drain.

Place both bunches of watercress on a serving dish or in a bowl. Garnish with lemon slices either in the center or off to one side.

Boiled Broccoli

4 cups broccoli flowerets
water

Place about ½ inch of water in a pot and bring to a boil. Add broccoli, cover, and reduce flame to medium-low. Simmer for 2–3 minutes or until broccoli is tender but still bright green and slightly crisp. Remove, drain, and place in a serving bowl.

Boiled Chinese Cabbage

4 cups Chinese cabbage, sliced diagonally into
    pieces about 1 inch wide
1 umeboshi plum
water

Place about 1 inch of water in a pot and add umeboshi plum. Bring to a boil. Add Chinese cabbage, cover, and reduce flame to medium-low. Simmer for 1–2 minutes so that cabbage remains crisp. Remove, drain, and place in a serving bowl. The umeboshi plum may be saved for use in other recipes.

Chinese-Style Vegetables

---

3 cups water
½ cup onions, cut into half-moons
3 shiitake mushrooms, soaked, stems
   removed, and sliced
½ cup carrots, cut into matchsticks
1 cup broccoli flowerets
1 cup Chinese cabbage, sliced diagonally into
   pieces about 1 inch wide
1½ tablespoons kuzu
tamari

Place water in a pot and bring to a boil. Add onions and shiitake and reduce flame to medium-low. Cover and simmer for 4–5 minutes. Add carrots and broccoli and simmer, covered, for 2–3 minutes. Add Chinese cabbage and simmer, covered, for 1 minute more.

To make sauce, dilute kuzu in 2–3 tablespoons of water. Reduce flame to low and add diluted kuzu, stirring constantly to prevent lumping. When kuzu becomes translucent and creamy, season vegetables with a little tamari to obtain a mild salt taste. Serve Chinese-Style Vegetables over croquettes, noodles, or plain rice, or as a vegetable side dish.

Boiled Red Radishes with
Umeboshi-Kuzu Sauce

---

2 cups water
4 shiso leaves
1 umeboshi plum
2 cups red radishes, trimmed
3 tablespoons kuzu
1 tablespoon sliced scallions or parsley

Place water, shiso leaves, umeboshi plum, and radishes in a pot and bring water to a boil. Cover, reduce flame to medium-low, and simmer until radishes are tender. Remove and drain radishes and shiso leaves, reserving cooking water. Set umeboshi plum aside. Place radishes in a shallow serving bowl. Chop shiso leaves and set aside.

Dilute kuzu in a few tablespoons of water and pour into cooking water. The water should be light red. Stir constantly to avoid lumping. When sauce becomes thick and creamy, remove from flame and pour over radishes. Place chopped shiso leaves in the center of the radishes. Sprinkle scallions or parsley on top for garnish, and serve.

Quickly Boiled Watercress and Carrots

---

1 carrot, thinly sliced on a diagonal
2 bunches of watercress
water

Place 1 inch of water in a pot and bring to a boil. Cook carrots for 50–60 seconds. Use a slotted spoon to remove carrots, leaving the water in the pot. Drain carrots in a colander. Simmer watercress for 50 seconds, stirring or mixing quickly to cook evenly. Remove watercress, drain, and place on cutting board. Slice into 2-inch pieces. Mix carrots and watercress in a serving bowl. Serve with Umeboshi-Sesame Dressing.

Watercress Sushi

---

4 bunches of watercress
4 sheets toasted nori (page 177)
8–12 shiso leaves
½ cup roasted sesame or sunflower seeds
    (page 191)

Place about 1 inch of water in a pot and bring to a boil. Boil watercress for about 50 seconds, stirring or mixing to cook evenly. Remove watercress, drain it, and rinse it under cold water to stop the cooking process and keep the bright green color. Using both hands, squeeze out excess water; set watercress on a plate.

Place a sheet of toasted nori on a bamboo sushi mat. Take 1 bunch of watercress and spread it evenly over the nori sheet. Cover about ¾ of the sheet, leaving 2 inches at the top edge and 1 inch at the bottom edge uncovered.

Take 2 or 3 shiso leaves and place them in a straight line across the watercress. Sprinkle about ⅛ cup of the sesame or sunflower seeds in a straight line on top of the shiso leaves.

Use both hands to roll the sushi mat into a cylinder shape, pressing mat firmly against nori and rice. When nori sheet is completely rolled up, wet the top edge lightly with water and press to seal edges tightly. Before unrolling sushi mat, squeeze gently to remove excess liquid.

Wet a sharp vegetable knife and slice nori roll in half. Wet knife again and slice each half into 4 equal sections (rounds), approximately 1 inch thick. You may need to wet knife slightly before making each cut. Repeat entire process with other sheets of nori.

Arrange sushi on an attractive platter with cut side facing up, and serve.

Steamed Broccoli

---

4 cups broccoli flowerets
water

Place about 1 inch of water in a pot. Set a steamer down inside the pot. Place broccoli in steamer, cover pot, and bring to a boil. Reduce flame to medium-low and steam broccoli several minutes, until it is tender but still firm and bright green. Remove and place in a serving bowl.

Steamed Kale

4 cups kale, sliced diagonally
water
tamari (optional)

Place about 1 inch of water in a pot. Set a steamer down inside the pot and bring water to a boil. Place kale in steamer. Cover, reduce flame to medium-low, and steam for 1–2 minutes. Sprinkle several drops of tamari on the kale and mix. Cover and steam for another minute or so, until kale is tender but slightly crisp and bright green. Remove and place in a serving dish.

Steamed Chinese Cabbage

4 cups Chinese cabbage, sliced into pieces
1–1½ inches wide
water

Place about 1 inch of water in a pot. Set a steamer down inside the pot and bring water to a boil. Add Chinese cabbage. Cover and steam for 2 minutes, so that cabbage is slightly crisp. Remove and place in a serving bowl.

Steamed Kale and Carrots

3 cups kale, stems and greens,
  sliced diagonally
1 cup carrots, thinly sliced on a diagonal
¼ cup roasted sunflower seeds (page 191)
water

Place about 2 inches of water in a pot. Set a bamboo steamer on top of the pot and bring water to a boil. Place carrots in steamer, cover, and steam for 3–4 minutes. Remove carrots and place in a serving bowl.

Make sure that the kale stems are sliced thinner than the leaves, so that they will cook evenly. Place stems in steamer, cover, and steam for 1 minute. Add kale greens and steam for 2–3 minutes. Remove steamed kale and mix in with carrots. Mix in roasted sunflower seeds, and serve.

Steamed Collard Greens

---

3 cups collard greens, thinly sliced
  on a diagonal
1 cup onions, cut into thin half-moons
water

Place about 1 inch of water in a pot. Set a steamer down inside the pot and bring water to a boil. Add onions and collard greens. Cover and reduce flame to medium-low. Steam for 2–3 minutes, until collards are tender and bright green. Remove and place in a serving bowl.

Kinpura Carrots and Burdock

---

1 cup burdock, cut into matchsticks or shaved
2 cups carrots, cut into matchsticks
dark sesame oil
water
tamari

Heat a small amount of dark sesame oil in a cast iron or stainless steel skillet. Sauté burdock over fairly high flame for 3–4 minutes. Place carrots on top of burdock, add several drops of water, and cover skillet. Reduce flame to medium-low. Simmer several minutes, until carrots and burdock are tender. Season with a little tamari and simmer 2–3 minutes longer. Remove cover and cook off any remaining liquid. Mix carrots and burdock, remove from flame, and place in a serving bowl.

Sautéed Burdock with Sesame Seeds

---

3 cups burdock, cut into matchsticks or shaved
½ cup sesame seeds
dark sesame oil
water
brown rice vinegar
tamari

Heat a small amount of dark sesame oil in a skillet. Place burdock in skillet and sauté over fairly high flame for 4–5 minutes. Add a few drops of water to lightly cover the bottom of the skillet. Cover and reduce flame to medium-low. Cook until burdock is tender. Remove cover and cook off any remaining liquid.

Dry-roast sesame seeds in a stainless steel skillet, until they are golden brown and release a nutty fragrance. Stir seeds back and forth constantly to keep them from burning. Place roasted seeds in a suribachi, and grind until they are about half crushed.

Mix in a few drops of brown rice vinegar and several drops of tamari. Add enough water to make a thick paste, and mix. Place burdock in with sesame seeds and mix to thoroughly coat burdock. Remove and place in a serving bowl.

Dried Daikon and Kombu

---

4 shiitake mushrooms, soaked,
    stems removed, and sliced
2 kombu strips, 6 inches long, soaked and
    thinly sliced
2 cups dried daikon, rinsed, soaked,
    and sliced
water (include daikon and shiitake soaking
    water)
dark sesame oil
tamari

Heat a small amount of dark sesame oil in a skillet. Add shiitake
and sauté for 3–4 minutes. Add kombu, set daikon on top of kombu, and add enough water to half cover the daikon. Cover skillet
and bring water to a boil. Reduce flame to medium-low and simmer
for 25–30 minutes. Season with a little tamari to obtain a mild salt
taste and continue to cook several minutes longer, until all liquid
has evaporated. Mix vegetables and place in a serving bowl.

Nishime Vegetables

---

1 kombu strip, 6 inches long, soaked and cut
    into 1-inch squares
1 piece daikon, 4–5 inches long, halved
    lengthwise and cut into half-moons 1 inch
    thick
1 cup butternut *or* buttercup squash, cut in
    1½-inch chunks
1 cup carrots, cut into chunks
pinch of sea salt
water
tamari

Place kombu in a heavy pot. Place daikon on top of kombu. Set
squash on top of daikon, and place carrots on top of squash. Add a
pinch of sea salt and about ½ inch of water. Cover pot and bring
water to a boil. Reduce flame to low and simmer until vegetables
are tender. Add a small amount of tamari and continue to simmer
until vegetables are soft and all liquid has evaporated. Mix
vegetables with kombu, remove, and place in a serving bowl.

Grated Daikon

---

1 piece daikon, 6–8 inches long
1 fresh parsley sprig or small
    daikon leaf
tamari

Grate daikon on a flat grater and place in a small serving dish. Place
3 or 4 drops of tamari in the center of the daikon and garnish with a
small sprig of fresh parsley or with a small daikon leaf to one side of
the dish. Serve each person 1 or 2 tablespoons.

Pickled Vegetables

Red Radish Pickles

10–12 red radishes, trimmed
¾ cup water
¼ cup umeboshi vinegar

Slice radishes into very thin rounds and place in a pickle press. Add
water and umeboshi vinegar. Place top on pickle press and screw
down. Let sit for at least 2–3 hours.

You may leave radishes in pickle press for as long as 1–2 days; the
longer you leave them, the saltier and stronger they become. If
pickles become too salty, simply rinse with cold water before
eating. If pickles are very salty, serve 2 or 3 slices to each person. If
pickles are mild, several pieces are fine. Red Radish Pickles will
keep for about 1 week in the refrigerator or in a cool place.

Rice Bran Pickles

---

4 cups rice bran (nuka)
1 piece daikon, 12–14 inches long,
     quartered lengthwise
1½ tablespoons sea salt
water

Place rice bran in a dry skillet. Stirring constantly to prevent burning, roast for several minutes over low flame until a nutty fragrance
is released. Remove from flame and allow to cool. When rice bran is
cool, place it in a large ceramic or wooden crock or keg. Mix in sea

salt and add enough cold water to form a very thick, slightly dry paste. Cut each piece of daikon in half, to obtain a total of 8 pieces, and place them in the keg, making sure that they are completely covered with rice bran paste. Cover the top of the crock or keg with clean cotton cheesecloth to keep dust out.

Let sit for 5–7 days in a fairly cool place. Mix ingredients daily to pickle evenly and prevent souring. After 5–7 days, remove pickles, rinse under cold water, and slice paper-thin. Arrange on a small serving dish or in a small bowl. Serve 2 or 3 slices to each person.

Broccoli Pickles

---

2 cups small broccoli flowerets
¾ cup water
¼ cup tamari
2 slices of fresh ginger

Place all ingredients in a pickle press or jar. Apply just enough pressure to hold the broccoli under the tamari-water solution. If you use a jar, take a smaller jar or a drinking cup that fits inside and press the pickles by setting a weight in that cup. Let sit for 2–3 days. If pickles are too salty, rinse with cold water before eating. These pickles will keep for about 1 week in a cool place.

Quick Cucumber Pickles

---

2 cups cucumbers, thinly sliced on a diagonal
2 tablespoons brown rice vinegar
½ teaspoon sea salt

Place all ingredients in a pickle press and mix thoroughly. Place top on pickle press and screw down. When water level rises to pressure plate, release pressure slightly and let sit for 2–3 hours. Remove, squeeze out excess liquid, and place pickles on a serving dish.

Chinese Cabbage Pickles

---

1 head Chinese cabbage
¼ cup sea salt (approximately)

Wash cabbage leaves by individually removing them from the head. Place in a colander to allow water to drain. When all water has drained off, the cabbage leaves are ready to use.

Sprinkle a thin layer of sea salt in the bottom of a ceramic crock or wooden keg. Layer whole cabbage leaves and salt in the keg or crock, alternating salt and cabbage. The bottom and top layers should always be salt. You may also place a strip of kombu at the bottom of the crock. The kombu absorbs water, adds minerals, and changes the taste of the pickles. On top of the first layer of salt, place a layer of leaves aligned in one direction. Add a thin layer of salt (several pinches are sufficient), and align a layer of leaves opposite in direction to the first layer. Repeat layering until all cabbage is used. Place a plate on top of the last layer of salt. Set several clean, heavy rocks on the plate to press the leaves down.

If water does not start to come out of the cabbage within 10–12 hours, more salt is needed. When water rises up to the level of the plate, remove some of the weight so that the level drops just below the plate. Check the water level every day and make sure that all is going well.

Pickles may be eaten after 3–4 days, or they may be left several days longer for a more sour taste. Rinse and slice before serving. Excess salt can be washed off by dipping pickles in warm water or soaking them for a short time. Store in a cool, dark place.

If the pickles begin to spoil at any point during the pickling process, add more salt or more pressure, and skim off the mold. It may be necessary to start again with fresh cabbage.

Onion Pickles

---

2 cups onions, cut into thin half-moons
1 cup water
½ cup tamari

Place all ingredients in a pickle press. Place top on pickle press and apply just enough pressure to hold onions under the tamari-water solution. Leave pickles for 1–2 days; the longer they sit, the saltier they will become. If they become too salty, rinse under cold water before eating. These pickles will keep for about 1 week in a cool place.

Sauerkraut

---

5 pounds cabbage
⅓ cup sea salt

Wash and finely shred cabbage. Place it in a wooden keg or ceramic crock and mix sea salt in very well. Place several clean rocks on top of a plate to press the cabbage. Cover with a piece of clean cheesecloth to keep dust out. Within 10 hours, the water level in the keg will rise up to or above the plate. If the level is above the plate, remove some of the weight to make the water recede. Keep sauerkraut in a cool, dark place for 1½–2 weeks. Check it every day to make sure all is going well. If mold begins to form on top, remove and discard it immediately.

When sauerkraut is ready, rinse it with cold water and place in a serving dish.

Daikon Pickles

---

2 cups daikon, cut into thin half-moons
1 teaspoon lemon peel, cut into thick
    matchsticks
¼ teaspoon sea salt

Place all ingredients in a pickle press and mix thoroughly. Place top on pickle press and screw down. Leave for 2–3 hours. Remove lemon peels and discard. Place the top back on, apply enough pressure to keep the water level just below the pressure plate, and let pickles sit for 1 day. Remove and place in a serving dish.

Cucumber Pickles

---

        10 cups water
        ⅓ cup sea salt
        12–15 cucumbers, quartered lengthwise
            (about 3 pounds)
        2 fresh dill sprigs

Place water and salt in a large crock or clean glass jar. Stir until salt dissolves. Add cucumbers and dill. Place clean cotton cheesecloth over the top of the crock or jar to allow air in and to keep dust out. Leave in a cool place for 2–3 days. Refrigerate and let sit 2–3 more days. Place on an attractive serving tray, and serve.

See also *Pressed Salad*, page 172.

Salads

Boiled Salad

        ½ cup onions, cut into thick half-moons
        1 cup kale, sliced into pieces about
            1½ inches wide
        ½ cup carrots, cut into thin half-moons
        1 cup cabbage, cut into 1-inch chunks
        water

Place about 1 inch of water in a pot and bring to a boil. Boil onions for about 1 minute. Use a slotted spoon or a pair of cooking chopsticks to remove onions, leaving the cooking water in the pot. Drain onions in a colander before placing in a large serving bowl. Boil kale in the same water for 1–2 minutes; remove and drain. Place in bowl with onions.

Then boil carrots in the same water for 1–2 minutes. Remove cooked carrots, drain, and mix in with kale and onions. Finally, cook the cabbage in the boiling water for about 2 minutes. Remove, drain, and mix in with other vegetables. Serve Boiled Salad plain or with dressing.

Boiled Salad with Tempeh

---

1 cup tempeh, cut into 1-inch cubes
2 slices of fresh ginger
½ cup carrots, thinly sliced on a diagonal
2 cups broccoli flowerets
1 cup cabbage, cut into 1-inch chunks
dark sesame oil
tamari
water

Heat a small amount of dark sesame oil in a skillet. Place tempeh and ginger in skillet and sauté for 3–4 minutes over fairly high flame. Add just enough water to cover the bottom of the skillet. Cover skillet and reduce flame to low. Simmer for 25–30 minutes.

Season with a little tamari to give a mild salt taste and continue to cook for 5–10 more minutes. Remove cover and cook off all remaining liquid. Place tempeh in a serving bowl and set ginger aside for use in other dishes.

Place 1 inch of water in a pot and bring to a boil. Add carrots. Cover and reduce flame to medium-low. Cook for 1–2 minutes. Use a slotted spoon to remove carrots, leaving the cooking water in the pot. Drain carrots in a colander before placing in serving bowl with tempeh. Cook broccoli in the same boiling water for 2–3 minutes, until tender, bright green, and slightly crisp. Remove broccoli, drain, and place in bowl with carrots and tempeh. Cook cabbage in the boiling water for 2–3 minutes. Remove, drain, and place in bowl with other ingredients. Mix and serve.

Watercress Salad

---

1 cup carrots, cut into matchsticks
3 bunches of watercress
water

Place 1 inch of water in a pot and bring to a boil. Simmer carrots for 1 minute. Use a slotted spoon to remove carrots, leaving the cooking water in the pot. Drain carrots in a colander before placing in a serving bowl. Cook watercress in the same boiling water for 50 seconds, stirring or mixing to cook evenly. Remove and drain. Toss to cool, or spread apart on a plate. Slice watercress into 2-inch slices and mix in with carrots. Serve with Umeboshi-Scallion Dressing.

Pressed Salad

---

2 cups Chinese cabbage, very thinly sliced
1 cup cucumber, sliced
½ cup red radishes, thinly sliced
¼ cup onions, cut into very thin half-moons
3 tablespoons brown rice vinegar
½ teaspoon sea salt

Place all ingredients in a pickle press and mix thoroughly to coat vegetables evenly with vinegar and salt. Place top on pickle press and screw down firmly. The salt causes the water in the vegetables to come out. When water level rises to the pressure plate, release pressure slightly to allow vegetables to absorb salt and vinegar. Let sit for 1–2 hours. Remove salad vegetables, squeeze out excess liquid, and place salad in a serving bowl.

Garden Salad

---

3 cups fresh iceberg or romaine lettuce,
    sliced or pulled apart
½ cup carrots, shredded or coarsely grated
½ cup red onions, cut into thin half-moons
¼ cup celery, thinly sliced on a diagonal
1 cucumber, unwaxed

Place lettuce, carrot, onion, and celery in a serving bowl and toss to mix evenly. With a fork, make straight grooves down the skin of an unwaxed cucumber, digging into skin only about $^1/_{16}$ inch. Slice cucumber into thin rounds and mix in with other salad ingredients. Serve with Umeboshi-Sunflower Dressing.

See also *Hijiki Salad*, page 176.

BEANS, BEAN PRODUCTS, AND SEA VEGETABLES

Fried Tempeh with Ginger

2 cups onions, cut into half-moons
1 pound tempeh, cut into 1-inch cubes
1 tablespoon juice from freshly grated ginger
dark sesame oil
water
tamari

Heat a small amount of dark sesame oil in a skillet. Sauté onions for 2–3 minutes over fairly high flame, stirring constantly. Add tempeh and sauté for 1–2 minutes. Add enough water to half cover onions and tempeh; add ginger juice and cover skillet. Reduce flame to medium-low and cook for 25 minutes. Season with a small amount of tamari and simmer several minutes longer. Remove cover, turn flame up slightly, and cook until all water has evaporated. Mix onions and tempeh together and place in a serving bowl.

Fried Tofu

1 pound fresh firm-style tofu
dark sesame oil
tamari

Slice tofu into pieces 3 inches long by 2 inches wide by ½ inch thick. Heat a small amount of dark sesame oil in a skillet. Set sliced tofu in skillet and pour 2 or 3 drops of tamari on top of each slice. Fry over medium-high flame for 2–3 minutes. Turn slices over and place 1 or 2 drops of tamari on top. Fry for 2–3 minutes. Turn over once more and fry for 1–2 minutes so that both sides are golden brown. Remove and arrange attractively on a platter. Garnish with a sprig of fresh parsley either in the center or off to one side of the platter.

Boiled Tempeh and Scallions

---

1 pound tempeh
1 tablespoon scallion roots (the white part and
   root hairs), finely chopped
2 cups scallions, sliced into 2-inch lengths
water
tamari

Slice tempeh into pieces 2 inches long by 1 inch wide by ½ inch thick. Heat ¼ cup water in a skillet. Add scallion roots and water-sauté over high flame for 2–3 minutes. Add tempeh and enough water to half cover tempeh. Bring to a boil. Cover, reduce flame to medium-low, and simmer for 25 minutes. Season with a little tamari, cover, and simmer for another 5 minutes or so. Add sliced scallions so that they sit on top of tempeh (do not mix). Cover and cook for 1–2 minutes, until scallions are tender and bright green. Remove cover, turn flame to high, and cook off any remaining liquid. Mix and place in a serving dish.

Scrambled Tofu

---

1 cup onions, diced
¼ cup burdock, cut into matchsticks
½ cup carrots, cut into matchsticks
1 pound fresh tofu
½ cup chopped parsley
dark sesame oil
tamari or sea salt

Heat a small amount of dark sesame oil in a skillet. Sauté onions over fairly high flame for 2–3 minutes. Layer burdock and carrots on top of onions. Crumble tofu on top. Cover, reduce flame to medium-low, and cook several minutes, until tofu is soft and fluffy and vegetables are tender. Season with a little tamari or sea salt and continue to cook, uncovered, until almost all liquid has evaporated. Mix in parsley and place in a serving bowl.

Broiled Tofu

---

1 pound fresh firm-style tofu
tamari

Slice tofu into pieces 3 inches long by 2 inches wide by ½ inch thick. Place on a cookie sheet and put 2 or 3 drops of tamari on each slice. Place in the broiler and broil until golden brown. Turn slices over, put 1 or 2 drops of tamari on top, and place back in the broiler. Broil for 2–3 minutes, until tofu is golden brown and very soft. Remove and arrange attractively on a serving platter.

Aduki Beans with Kombu and Squash

---

1 kombu strip, 6–8 inches long, soaked and cut
    into 1-inch squares
1 cup buttercup squash *or* Hokkaido
    pumpkin, cut into 2-inch chunks
1 cup aduki beans, soaked 6–8 hours
water
sea salt

Place kombu in a pot and set squash on top. Place aduki beans on top of squash. Add just enough water to cover squash but not beans. Bring to a boil, cover, and reduce flame to medium-low. Simmer 1½–2 hours or until beans are fairly soft. Season with a little sea salt (¼ teaspoon per cup of beans at most). Simmer another half hour or until beans are very creamy and much of the remaining liquid is gone. Place in a serving bowl and serve.

Sea Vegetables

Hijiki Salad

---

2 cups hijiki, soaked and sliced
1 cup onions, cut into half-moons
½ cup carrots, cut into matchsticks
½ cup celery, thinly sliced on a diagonal
¼ cup roasted sunflower seeds (page 191)
water
tamari

Place about ½ inch of water in a saucepan and bring to a boil. Add hijiki and several drops of tamari. Cover saucepan, reduce flame to medium-low, and simmer for 15–20 minutes. Remove, drain, and place hijiki in a serving bowl.

Place 1 inch of water in a pot and bring to a boil. Add onions and boil for 1 minute. Use a slotted spoon to remove onions, leaving the cooking water in the pot. Drain onions in a colander before placing in bowl with hijiki. Boil carrots in the same water for 1–2 minutes. Remove, drain, and place in bowl with hijiki and onions. Next boil celery in the same water for 1 minute. Remove, drain, and place in bowl with hijiki and vegetables. Mix thoroughly; add roasted sunflower seeds and mix again. Serve plain or with tofu or umeboshi dressing.

Arame with Carrots and Onions

---

2 cups arame, washed and drained
1 cup onions, cut into half-moons
1 cup carrots, cut into matchsticks
dark sesame oil
water
tamari

Heat a small amount of dark sesame oil in a skillet. Sauté arame for 2-3 minutes. Set onions and carrots on top of arame and add enough water to half cover arame. Add 3 or 4 drops of tamari, cover skillet, and reduce flame to medium-low. Simmer for about 25-30 minutes. Season with a little more tamari for a mild salt taste and continue cooking until all remaining liquid is gone. Place in a serving dish.

Toasted Nori

---

1 sheet nori

To toast nori, turn flame to high. Hold nori sheet about 10 inches above flame with inside fold facing down (toward flame). Rotate nori sheet above flame until its color changes from black to bright green. Remove from flame.

To make nori strips, cut toasted nori sheet crosswise. Cut each section crosswise again, to create 4 large strips. Then, across the width of these large strips, cut thin strips about 2 inches long by ¼ inch wide.

Serve toasted nori strips with grated daikon or mochi, or as a garnish for soups or noodles.

SOUPS

Lentil Soup

---

1 kombu strip, 6 inches long, soaked and cut
   into ½-inch squares
1 cup onions, diced
1 cup celery, diced
1 cup green lentils
5-6 cups water
1 cup whole wheat elbow noodles or shells
¼ cup chopped parsley
sea salt

Place kombu, onions, celery, lentils, and water in a pot. Cover and bring to a boil. Reduce flame to medium-low and simmer for about 45 minutes. Season with a little sea salt, add the uncooked noodles, and simmer for several minutes more, uncovered, until noodles are tender. Place soup in individual serving bowls and garnish with a little chopped parsley.

Chick Pea Soup

---

1 cup chick peas, soaked 6–8 hours
1 kombu strip, 6–8 inches long, soaked and cut
   into 1-inch squares
1 cup onions, diced
5 cups water
sea salt

Place chick peas, kombu, and onions in a pressure cooker. Add water and place cover on pressure cooker. Turn flame to high and bring cooker up to pressure. Reduce flame to medium-low and cook for 1 hour.

Remove cooker from flame and allow pressure to come down. Remove cover and season with a little sea salt for a mild taste. Simmer several minutes longer. Place soup in individual serving bowls and garnish with chopped scallions or parsley.

Miso Soup

---

5 cups water
4 or 5 shiitake mushrooms, soaked,
   stems removed, and sliced
1 kombu strip, 6 inches long
4–5 teaspoons puréed barley (mugi) miso
   (adjust to taste)
1 cup fresh snow peas, stems removed

Place water, shiitake, and kombu in a pot and bring to a boil. Cover and reduce flame to medium-low. Simmer for about 10 minutes. Remove kombu, slice very thin, and place back in water. Reduce flame to very low; add puréed miso and snow peas and simmer 2–3 minutes longer. Place soup in individual serving bowls, and serve.

French Onion Soup

4–5 cups onions, thinly sliced on a diagonal
4 or 5 shiitake mushrooms, soaked,
    stems removed, and sliced
5 cups water
2 slices whole wheat sourdough bread,
    sliced into 1-inch cubes
¼ cup chopped scallions, chives, or parsley
dark sesame oil
tamari

Heat a small amount of dark sesame oil in a pot. Sauté onions 3–4 minutes, until onions are translucent. Add sliced shiitake mushrooms and sauté for another 1–2 minutes.

Add water and bring to a boil. Cover pot and reduce flame to medium-low; simmer for 30 minutes or until onions are very soft. Season with a small amount of tamari for a mild-tasting soup.

Heat 1 inch of sesame oil in a skillet. When oil is hot, add bread cubes and deep-fry until golden brown. Remove and drain on clean paper towels.

Place soup in individual serving bowls and garnish each serving with several deep-fried bread cubes and some chopped scallions, chives, or parsley. A few strips of toasted nori may be used in addition.

Instead of bread cubes, you may use 1-inch squares of baked, toasted, or deep-fried mochi for garnish.

Watercress Soup
---

5 cups water
1 kombu strip, 4 inches long, soaked
4 shiitake mushrooms, soaked,
    stems removed, and sliced
½ cup tofu, sliced into ¼-inch cubes
½ bunch of watercress

Place water, kombu, and shiitake in a pot and bring to a boil. Cover and reduce flame to medium-low. Simmer for 10 minutes. Remove kombu and set aside for use in other dishes. Add tofu and miso, reduce flame to very low, and simmer for 2–3 minutes. Place 2 or 3 sprigs of watercress in each individual serving bowl and pour the hot soup over it. The heat from the soup will be enough to properly cook the watercress. Serve soup immediately after placing it in bowls.

Puréed Squash Soup

5–6 cups buttercup squash *or* Hokkaido
    pumpkin, cut into chunks
4–5 cups water
1 sheet nori, toasted and cut into thin strips
    (page 177)
¼ cup chopped scallions or parsley
sea salt

Place squash, water, and a small pinch of sea salt in a pot. Cover and bring to a boil. Reduce flame to medium-low and simmer for several minutes, until squash is very soft and tender. Place squash and cooking water in a hand food mill and purée to a smooth, creamy consistency. Return puréed squash to pot and bring back to a boil. Reduce flame to low, season with a little sea salt, and simmer for about 10 minutes. Place soup in individual serving bowls and garnish with chopped scallions or parsley and several strips of toasted nori.

Miso Soup with Wakame and Daikon

---

5 cups water
2 cups daikon, quartered and thinly sliced
    on a diagonal
3 shiitake mushrooms, soaked,
    stems removed, and sliced
¼ cup wakame, washed, soaked, and sliced
4–5 teaspoons puréed barley (mugi) miso
    (adjust to taste)
¼ cup chopped scallions

Place water in a pot and bring to a boil. Add daikon and shiitake
mushrooms. Reduce flame to medium-low, cover, and simmer for
3–5 minutes, until daikon is tender. Add wakame and simmer for
2–3 minutes longer. Reduce flame to very low, season with puréed
miso for a mild taste, and simmer 2–3 minutes more. Place soup in
individual serving bowls and garnish with chopped scallions.

Seitan Barley Soup

---

1 kombu strip, 4 inches long, soaked and
    cut into ½-inch squares
¼ cup chopped parsley or scallions
¼ cup shiitake or regular mushrooms, sliced
1 cup onions, diced
¼ cup celery, diced
½ cup carrots, diced
¼ cup burdock, diced
¼ cup barley, soaked 6–8 hours
1 cup cooked seitan, cut into 1-inch cubes
    (page 151)
5 cups water
1 tablespoon finely chopped parsley stems or
    scallion roots (the white bottom part
    and root hairs)
tamari

Place kombu and parsley stems or scallion roots in a large pot. Layer shiitake, onions, celery, carrots, burdock, and barley (in that order) on top. Place cooked seitan on top of barley. Add water and bring to a boil. Cover and reduce flame to medium-low. Simmer for about 1 hour, until barley is very soft. Season with a little tamari and continue to simmer over low flame until soup is very soft and creamy. Place soup in individual serving bowls and garnish with chopped parsley or scallions.

Clear Broth

---

1 kombu strip, 4 inches long, soaked
5 cups water
½ cup celery, thinly sliced on a diagonal
2 cups Chinese cabbage, sliced diagonally
   into 1-inch pieces
sea salt
chopped scallions

Place kombu and water in a pot and bring to a boil. Cover, reduce flame to medium-low, and simmer for about 10 minutes. Remove kombu and set aside for future use. Add celery and cook for 1 minute. Add Chinese cabbage and cook for 2 minutes. Season with a little sea salt and simmer 2 minutes more. Place broth in individual serving bowls and garnish with chopped scallions.

Miso-Squash Soup

---

5 cups water
1 cup onions, cut into half-moons
2 cups acorn squash, cut into 1-inch chunks
½ cup wakame, washed, soaked, and sliced
4–5 teaspoons puréed barley (mugi) miso
   (adjust to taste)
¼ cup chopped scallions

Place water in a pot and bring to a boil. Add onions and squash. Cover pot and reduce flame to medium-low. Simmer for several minutes, until squash is tender. Add wakame and simmer for 2–3 minutes. Reduce flame to very low and add puréed miso for a mild taste. Place soup in individual serving bowls and garnish with chopped scallions.

SUPPLEMENTARY FOODS

Condiments

Gomashio

1⅓ tablespoons sea salt
1 cup black or tan sesame seeds

Place sea salt in a stainless steel skillet and roast over medium-low flame for several minutes, constantly stirring back and forth. Place sea salt in a suribachi and grind to a fine powder.

Heat a dry stainless steel skillet and place washed sesame seeds in it. Dry-roast seeds for several minutes, constantly stirring back and forth to roast evenly. When seeds give off a nutty fragrance and begin to pop, remove from flame and place in suribachi with ground sea salt. Grind in a slow circular motion until sesame seeds are about half crushed. Remove and allow to cool. When gomashio is cool, store in an airtight glass container. Sprinkle a small amount of this condiment on rice or other grain dishes.

Nori Condiment

---

5 sheets nori
water
tamari

Pull the nori apart into approximately 1-inch pieces and place in a saucepan. Pour a mixture of equal parts water and tamari over the nori to just cover it. Bring to a boil, reduce flame to low, cover, and simmer until most of the liquid is gone. Season with additional tamari to create a slightly salty taste. Serve each person 1–2 teaspoons of this condiment with rice or other grains.

Dressings, Butters and Spreads

Tofu Dressing

---

1 small onion, grated
¼ cup umeboshi vinegar *or*
    4 umeboshi plums, pitted
1 pound fresh tofu, drained
1 tablespoon tamari
½ cup chopped scallions or
    chives
½ cup water

Place onion and umeboshi vinegar or plums in a suribachi. If you use plums, grind to a smooth paste (with onion in suribachi). Purée tofu in a hand food mill. Place puréed tofu in suribachi and grind to a smooth consistency. Add tamari, scallions or chives, and water. Purée and place in an attractive serving dish. Place a tablespoon or so of dressing on top of Boiled Salad or Hijiki Salad, or use as a spread on bread, crackers, or rice cakes.

Umeboshi-Sunflower Dressing

---

2 umeboshi plums, pitted
¼ cup chopped scallions or chives
½ cup water
¼ cup roasted sunflower seeds (see page 191),
    chopped

Place plums in a suribachi and grind to a smooth paste. Add scallions or chives and grind for 2 minutes. Add water and sunflower seeds. Mix and serve over your favorite salad.

Umeboshi-Scallion Dressing

---

3 umeboshi plums, pitted
4 tablespoons tahini
¼ cup chopped scallions
1¼ cups water

Place umeboshi in a suribachi and grind to a smooth paste. Add tahini and grind again. Add scallions and water, mix to a smooth consistency, and serve over your favorite salad.

Umeboshi-Sesame Dressing

½ cup roasted sesame seeds (page 191)
¼ cup umeboshi vinegar
¾ cup water
¼ cup chopped scallions

Place roasted sesame seeds in a suribachi and grind until half crushed. Add vinegar, water, and scallions. Grind for 1–2 minutes. Serve over your favorite salad.

Onion Butter

---

10 cups onions, diced
pinch of sea salt
dark sesame oil
water

Heat a small amount of dark sesame oil in a heavy pot. Sauté onions for several minutes over medium-low flame, until they become translucent. Stir often to sauté onions evenly.

Add a pinch of sea salt and just enough water to cover the top of the onions. Cover pot and bring water to a boil. Reduce flame to low and simmer for several hours so that the onions become dark brown and very sweet. There should not be any liquid left and the onions should be almost melted. If necessary, add very small amounts of water occasionally during the cooking process to keep onions from burning.

When onion butter is ready, allow it to cool completely. Use immediately on bread or rice cakes, or place in a glass jar with a lid. Store either in the refrigerator or in a cool place.

Fish and Seafood

Baked Sole with Rice

---

1 cup onions, diced
½ cup celery, diced
4 cups pressure-cooked or boiled brown rice
¼ cup chopped parsley
2–3 pounds fresh fillet of sole
½ cup tamari
½ cup water
1 teaspoon fresh grated ginger
dark sesame oil
several lemon wedges

Heat a small amount of dark sesame oil in a skillet. Sauté onions and celery for 2–3 minutes. Place sautéed vegetables in a bowl with rice and parsley, and mix well. Transfer mixture to a casserole dish.

Mix tamari, water, and ginger together. Place sole in a shallow bowl or dish and pour tamari-water-ginger mixture over it. Let sole marinate for 30–45 minutes. Place marinated sole evenly on top of rice in casserole dish. Cover casserole and bake at 350° F for approximately 30 minutes or until fish becomes tender. Remove casserole cover and bake another 5 minutes. Sprinkle a little chopped parsley over fish and serve with several lemon wedges for garnish.

Ginger-Broiled Scallops

---

2 pounds fresh scallops
1 tablespoon fresh grated ginger
½ cup water
¼ cup tamari
⅛ cup sake (rice wine; optional)
2 fresh parsley sprigs

Clean scallops and place in a bowl. Mix ginger, water, tamari, and sake together and pour over scallops. Marinate for 15–20 minutes. Place marinated scallops on a baking sheet and broil for 5–10 minutes or until very tender. Do not broil too long, as they will become tough. Place broiled scallops in a serving dish and garnish with fresh parsley sprigs.

Desserts and Snacks

Raisin-Nut Cookies

---

3 cups rolled oats
¼ teaspoon sea salt
1½ cups whole wheat pastry flour
1 cup raisins
½ cup chopped almonds
½ cup chopped walnuts
3 tablespoons corn oil
1 cup barley malt
1 cup water

Mix rolled oats, sea salt, flour, raisins, and nuts together. Add oil and mix again. Add barley malt and mix thoroughly. Add water to make a thick batter. Place spoonfuls of batter about 1½ inches apart on oiled cookie sheets and press down to form cookies. If cookies are too thick, they will not cook thoroughly. Bake at 375° F for 25–30 minutes or until golden brown. This recipe will yield between 1 and 2 dozen cookies.

Blueberry Couscous Cake

2½ cups apple juice *or* water
½ cup raisins
2 cups couscous
pinch of sea salt

Topping

1 cup water
¼ cup barley malt
pinch of sea salt
3 cups fresh blueberries
2–3 tablespoons kuzu, diluted
    in a few tablespoons of water

Place apple juice or water in a pot. Add sea salt and raisins. Bring to a boil. Cover, reduce flame to medium-low, and simmer for about 10 minutes. Add couscous, cover, and simmer for 3–5 minutes. Turn off flame and let couscous sit, covered, for about 10 minutes. The heat in the pot will cook the couscous thoroughly. After 10 minutes or so, remove couscous and place it in a glass or ceramic cake pan.

To make topping, place water, barley malt, sea salt, and blueberries in a saucepan and bring to a boil. Reduce flame to low and add diluted kuzu. Stir constantly to prevent lumping. Simmer for 2–3 minutes and remove from flame.

Press couscous down firmly with a rice paddle before adding topping. Pour topping over cake, spreading blueberries evenly. Set aside and allow to cool before serving.

Applesauce

---

    2 cups water
    8–10 apples, peeled and sliced
    ¼ cup barley malt (optional)
    pinch of sea salt

Place water, apples, barley malt, and sea salt in a pot and bring to a boil. Reduce flame to low and simmer until apples are soft. Purée apples and cooking water in a hand food mill. For sweeter applesauce, cook a little longer so that the sauce becomes thick. Applesauce cooked without barley malt makes a good breakfast dish.

Stewed Pears

---

    5 or 6 pears, sliced
    pinch of sea salt
    4 cups water
    ½ cup raisins
    4–5 tablespoons kuzu, diluted in several
       tablespoons of water

Place pears, salt, water, and raisins in a pot and bring to a boil. Reduce flame to low and cover pot. Simmer for several minutes, until pears are soft. Add diluted kuzu, stirring to prevent lumping. Simmer 2–3 minutes and serve.

Apple-Raisin Kanten

---

    4 apples, sliced
    1 quart apple juice
    pinch of sea salt
    ½ cup raisins
    5–6 tablespoons agar-agar flakes

Place apples, apple juice, salt, and raisins in a pot. Stir in agar-agar flakes and bring to a boil. Reduce flame to low and simmer for several minutes, until apples are soft. Pour liquid and apples into a dish or mold. Refrigerate or keep in a cool place until jelled. This will take about an hour or so. If the kanten is hard, slice into squares and serve. If it has a softer consistency, spoon into individual dessert bowls.

Couscous Cake with Pear Sauce

2½ cups apple juice
2 cups couscous
pinch of sea salt

Topping
5 or 6 pears, peeled and sliced
pinch of sea salt
1 cup water

Place apple juice and a pinch of sea salt in a pot and bring to a boil. Reduce flame to low and add couscous. Cover and simmer for 2–3 minutes. Turn off flame and let couscous sit, covered, for several minutes.

Place couscous in a glass or ceramic cake pan and press down firmly and evenly.

To make pear sauce for topping, place pears, salt, and water in a pot and bring to a boil. Reduce flame, cover, and simmer for 4–5 minutes, until pears are soft. Purée in a hand food mill. Slice cake and spoon pear sauce over it while serving.

Roasted Nuts and Tamari Roasted Nuts

Raw almonds, walnuts, peanuts, and chestnuts are especially good roasted in the shell. Place whole nuts on a cookie sheet and roast in 350° F oven for 10–12 minutes. If you use shelled nuts, they will cook faster.

To make tamari roasted nuts, simply sprinkle a mixture of equal parts tamari and water over shelled nuts towards the end of cooking.

Roasted Seeds

Wash tan or black sesame seeds, hulled sunflower seeds, squash seeds, or green pumpkin seeds. Heat a skillet and dry-roast each variety separately over medium-low flame. Stir constantly to prevent burning and to roast seeds evenly.

Tan sesame seeds and sunflower seeds will turn golden brown and begin to pop after 5 minutes or so; pumpkin seeds are ready when they turn golden brown. Season seeds with a small amount of tamari, if desired.

Fresh acorn squash seeds may be roasted in the oven like nuts. They will turn golden brown.

Roasted Grains and Beans

Brown rice, sweet brown rice, barley, and rye can be dry-roasted for use as a snack. Soak grains for 24 hours prior to roasting. Heat a dry skillet and separately roast each type of grain until it turns golden brown and releases a nutty fragrance. Stir constantly to keep grain from burning. Wheatberries may be roasted in the same way for use in recipes such as Pressure-Cooked Brown Rice and Wheatberries (page 143), but they are not generally recommended as a snack food.

Dry-roasted black soybeans make a particularly good snack. Soak soybeans for 4–6 hours and dry-roast as described above. They are ready when the skin starts to split and the beans are brown inside. While beans are very hot, stir in a few drops of tamari, if desired, and continue cooking until the moisture steams off. Dried green peas may be dry-roasted in the same way; they are ready when the skin begins to split and the peas are thoroughly heated.

Roasted chick peas, aduki beans, and other beans are not generally recommended as a snack, as they can be difficult to digest, but they may be ground for use in home-made grain coffee.

Beverages

Bancha Tea

---

1 quart water
1–2 tablespoons bancha twigs

Place water and twigs in a teapot and bring to a boil. Reduce flame to low and simmer for 5–10 minutes. For milder-tasting tea, simmer for 3–4 minutes. (Children may enjoy tea brewed to this strength.) For strong tea, simmer for 10–15 minutes. Bancha tea is good any time of day, especially after meals.

Grain Coffee

---

1 teaspoon prepared grain coffee
1 cup boiling water

Prepared grain coffee is available at most natural foods stores. Place 1 teaspoonful in a cup and pour hot water over it. Stir and drink. If you use home-made grain coffee, adjust the amounts to taste.

Amasake Drink

Amasake

4 cups sweet brown rice
8 cups water
½ cup koji
⅛ teaspoon sea salt

Wash sweet rice and soak overnight in 8 cups of water. Place rice (and water) in pressure cooker. Place cover on pressure cooker, turn flame to high, and bring cooker up to pressure. Reduce flame to medium-low, place a flame deflector under cooker, and pressure cook for 30 minutes. Remove cooker from flame and allow pressure to come down. Let rice cool for 45 minutes.

Place rice in a glass bowl and mix in koji. Cover with a clean towel and set aside to ferment for 6–8 hours. Mix several times during the fermentation process to make sure that koji dissolves.

Place fermented rice in a pot. Add sea salt and bring to a boil (boiling stops the fermentation process). As soon as mixture starts to bubble, remove from flame and allow to cool.

Store amasake in a covered glass jar in the refrigerator. Use as a sweetener or in making Amasake Drink. For variety, you may use brown rice, millet, or barley in this recipe.

Amasake Drink

½ cup amasake
½ cup water

Place amasake and water in a blender and blend to a creamy consistency. Amasake drink may be served hot with ginger, or with a teaspoon of grain coffee stirred in. It may also be enjoyed cool.

15

At Home and on the Road

Eating at restaurants, entertaining, and traveling can be a healthful and enjoyable part of the macrobiotic lifestyle. This chapter offers a number of practical ideas that will help you in following the macrobiotic diet, wherever you may be.

Chances are that there is a meal for you in the kitchen of any restaurant if you know how to ask for it. "Without cheese, no dressing, meatless, no sauce, broiled or steamed instead of fried," are all requests that are becoming increasingly common these days. In fact, you can ask your waiter or waitress to tell you about ingredients, additives, and the way the food is cooked before you place your order. After all, you are paying for your meal, and restaurateurs want their customers to be happy. Be creative and bold enough to ask for what you want, and your meal will probably exceed your expectations.

Unfortunately, most restaurants use sugar, common salt, black pepper, eggs, cheese, milk, and a number of chemical additives in their dishes. Certainly many cafeterias, fast food establishments, "family" restaurants, and even some "health food" eateries are not the best choice. A local ethnic restaurant where some vegetarian foods are served is probably your best bet. Unless, of course, there is a macrobiotic restaurant in your area, or a natural foods restaurant that serves macrobiotic dishes.

At Italian restaurants, soup, vegetables, pasta, salad, and baked or broiled fish are usually available without meat or tomato sauce. Most Chinese and Japanese restaurants serve steamed fish, vegetables, and rice. Requests for brown rice and "no MSG" can usually be accommodated.

Seafood restaurants are good too, especially if they serve freshly caught fish and cook it without too many trimmings. Fried fish, along with other fried foods, are best avoided, because restaurants generally use lard (animal fat) for frying. With dinner in a seafood restaurant, you can usually get rice or salad, and cooked vegetables.

Greek, Middle Eastern, Indian, and Mexican restaurants usually serve one or more vegetarian grain and bean dishes. But in the case of the latter two, make sure you ask them to forego use of chili or curry, if possible. In any restuarant, it is best to make sure that vegetable oils, and not lard, are used in cooking.

ENTERTAINING

When you prepare a full course macrobiotic meal for friends, it will most certainly be tasty and healthful. Start with an appetizer, and follow with soup or salad. Serve fish with whole grains and vegetables for an entree. Dessert can be a piece of Couscous Cake with Pear Sauce. Bancha tea or grain coffee will complete the meal.

If you plan to dine with friends, you may want to tell them you don't eat meat, and perhaps offer to bring some home-cooked food for them to enjoy.

BRINGING LUNCH TO WORK

People who work outside the home frequently eat lunch out on weekdays. If you can find a restaurant where you can go for an occasional macrobiotic or natural foods lunch, you are fortunate. Nevertheless, on a day-to-day-basis, it is best to bring lunch to work with you.

Macrobiotic meals are quite portable. If you buy a one- or two-cup size wide-mouth insulated container such as a Thermos, you can transport whole grains, soups, stews, and beans. If these are warmed before you leave for work, the container will keep them warm. You may also choose to bring rice balls, cooked vegetables, salad, pickles, and a dessert such as granola or couscous cake. In addition, you may wish to bring in a snack such as rice cakes, raisins, dried apples, or roasted nuts or seeds, along with an insulated container of bancha tea.

Tasty and convenient sandwiches may be made with seitan, tempeh, or tofu and sliced cooked vegetables on sourdough or pita bread, with lettuce and pickles. The idea is to include some kind of whole grain, as well as something raw or pickled to lighten the meal. Leftovers from dinner the night before make especially good lunch meals. You may also want to get a teapot to brew fresh bancha tea at the office.

IN THE AIR

Fortunately, the airlines are on their best behavior since competition has made it necessary for them to do a little extra to get your business. As long as you call one day in advance of your flight, you can generally order the type of food you want on board. You may be able to order brown rice, miso soup, a bean dish, oatmeal, wild rice, or steamed vegetables. Beware of the "standard" vegetarian meal, as it usually comes filled with eggs, salt, and sugar, all floating in butter and topped with cheese. Your best bet is to call ahead to find out exactly what's available.

Just in case of a mishap, you can bring along a travel bag with an assortment of home-made sushi, rice balls, steamed and pickled vegetables, sourdough bread, powdered miso soup (available packaged—just pour the contents into a cup of hot water), and maybe a few home-made cookies and some bancha tea bags.

It is a good idea to eat less than usual when you travel. You will have more energy when you arrive at your destination, and feel better too.

ON THE ROAD

When you travel by car, you have more control over your food. If you bring a small cutting board, a sharp knife, several bowls, utensils, a small gas cooker (camping type with two burners), two or three pots, a couple of wooden spoons, and a cooler chest with refreezable ice cubes (these can be placed in a motel ice chest if you stop overnight), you won't have to dine out at all. For food, you will need some quick-cooking grains such as roasted rice or barley, rice cream, couscous, cornmeal, bulghur, and oatmeal; lentils, aduki, split peas and other quick-cooking beans; and sea vegetables, miso, tamari soy sauce, noodles, bancha tea, snacks, sourdough bread, and tortillas. You can store fresh vegetables and fruits, fish, amasake, tofu, tempeh, and other staples in a cooler, and replenish supplies along the way. If you're planning to stop at motels, try to get a unit with a kitchen so that you can thoroughly clean all of your equipment, make some rice balls, bake some bread, and prepare a meal or two.

If you plan to be on the road for an extended journey, prepare ahead of time by contacting the East West Foundation or the *East West Journal* for a list of natural foods stores and restaurants along your route. If you are in a city or town you can always look in the Yellow Pages under ''health'' to find suppliers of natural and macrobiotic foods. In many cases, local restaurants will also be listed. If not, call one of the health food stores and ask if they can recommend a local restaurant.

Spending a little extra time in preparation will make the trip smoother, keep you healthier, and save you money. Of course, you may have to go out of your way a bit to find alternatives, but as so many people have discovered, you will probably meet others with common interests, sample some tasty vegetarian meals, and stock up on supplies. When you return home, you will know that it was worth it.

Epilogue

The natural world nourishes, supports, and sustains plant, animal, and human life. We, in turn, are to care for it with our utmost respect. A disregard for the natural world leads to plundering of the earth's resources and pollution of its atmosphere and water. A renewed commitment to the preservation of biological life and to the natural harmony between humans and nature can help us to resolve these and other problems that threaten our wholeness and our very survival.

At the very heart of the larger problems facing humanity is a fragmented and dualistic view of life. In the dualistic view, we see a hostile world: a struggle between good and bad, sickness and health, and love and hate. This fundamental division of thought underlies all of our economic, educational, scientific, and political institutions.

Macrobiotic theory is based on unity and wholeness, not division. The macrobiotic view recognizes that nature attempts to maintain harmony and balance. Health is seen as a natural result of balanced thinking, living, and eating. Societal health results when the members of an entire society live in harmony with the natural world.

The macrobiotic view that all life in the universe is a unified, orderly system controlled by definite natural laws makes each person acutely aware of his or her role as creator and shaper not only of individual lives, but also of the whole of life on earth. With the power that comes from this knowledge, we can consciously bring about the level of energy, variety of experience, and quality of life that we desire.

Macrobiotics states that eating natural, wholesome food is the first step towards better health and quality of life. While balanced exercise and activity strengthen and energize the body, self-reflection brings knowledge of our thoughts and desires, helping us to understand ourselves and the world around us. With these beginnings, the macrobiotic way can lead to a peaceful, cooperative, and loving world.

Appendix A

Nutritional Analysis of a Typical Macrobiotic Daily Menu Compared with the U.S. RDAs

Throughout this book we have discussed the key nutrients supplied by the macrobiotic diet. In the chart that follows, this information is summarized and compared with the U.S. Recommended Daily Allowances (RDAs) for adults. The results of the analysis show that the macrobiotic diet more than satisfies the RDAs for all the necessary nutrients.

The most important factor in ensuring that all the key nutrients are supplied every day by the macrobiotic diet is the use of a variety of the recommended foods, and the proper cooking of them. When eaten in the suggested proportion with one another (see Chapter 1), these foods will supply enough high-quality nutrients to maintain excellent health and vitality.

ESTIMATED NUTRITIONAL ANALYSIS
OF A TYPICAL MACROBIOTIC MENU*

The following menu is for one person for one day.

Food	Amount	Calories	Protein	Fat	Carbohydrate
Measurement Units				Grams	
BREAKFAST					
Oatmeal	2 cups	260	10.0	2.0	46.0
Whole Wheat Sourdough Bread with Apple Butter	2 slices; 2 tablespoons	210	5.1	1.2	43.7
Bancha Tea	1 cup	2	—	trace	.4
LUNCH					
Cucumber Sushi **Tempeh-Sauerkraut Sushi**	¼ recipe ¼ recipe	420	17.8	6.2	65.4
Boiled Salad with Tofu Dressing	1 serving	86	7.3	1.6	12.9
Bancha Tea	1 cup	2	—	trace	.4
SNACK					
Roasted Almonds and Sunflower Seeds with Raisins	½ cup	318	8.1	16.0	39.0

Note: A dash signifies a lack of reliable data for a constituent believed to be present in a measurable amount.

Source:
*Estimated nutritional content of this macrobiotic menu is based on *USDA Composition of Foods Handbook No. 8.*

Calcium	Phosphorus	Iron	Sodium	Potassium	Vitamin A	Vitamin B$_1$ (thiamine)	Vitamin B$_2$ (riboflavin)	Niacin	Vitamin C (ascorbic acid)
Milligrams					I.U.		Milligrams		
44	232	3.0	344	292	0	.38	.10	.4	0
54	150	1.8	257	245	trace	.18	.06	1.6	trace
—	—	trace	—	—	—	—	—	—	—
61	177	12.1	497	246	800	.41	.34	6.9	25
107	77	5.8	166	616	1055	.16	.18	1.3	68
—	—	trace	—	—	—	—	—	—	—
88	279	3.1	17	594	16	1.10	.30	1.5	trace

ESTIMATED NUTRITIONAL ANALYSIS
OF A TYPICAL MACROBIOTIC MENU*—*Continued*

Food	Amount	Calories	Protein	Fat	Carbohydrate
Measurement Units			Grams		
DINNER					
Miso Soup	1 bowl	59	3.0	0.7	7.7
Baked Sole with Rice	1 serving	396	21.5	9.5	70.4
Grated Daikon	¼ cup	5	.3	—	1.0
Quickly Boiled Watercress and Carrots with Umeboshi-Scallion Dressing	1 serving	81	3.3	2.6	8.5
Couscous Cake with Pear Sauce	1 serving	287	2.6	.4	65.7
Grain Coffee	1 cup	—	—	—	—
TOTALS		2126	79.0	40.2	361.1

Note: A dash signifies a lack of reliable data for a constituent believed to be present in a measurable amount.

Source:
*Estimated nutritional content of this macrobiotic menu is based on *USDA Composition of Foods Handbook No. 8.*

Calcium	Phosphorus	Iron	Sodium	Potassium	Vitamin A	Vitamin B$_1$ (thiamine)	Vitamin B$_2$ (riboflavin)	Niacin	Vitamin C (ascorbic acid)
Milligrams					I.U.		Milligrams		
148	96	6.9	349	205	83	.50	.70	.4	22
66	378	2.8	361	525	140	.25	.11	6.6	trace
9	6	.2	150	195	3	—	—	—	10
264	82	1.8	165	350	12,662	.06	.02	1.0	80
18	62	1.8	254	398	30	.03	.04	.6	31
—	—	—	—	—	—	—	—	—	—
859	1539	39.3	2560	3666	14,789	3.07	1.85	20.3	236

SUMMARY—
TYPICAL MACROBIOTIC MENU
TOTALS COMPARED TO THE 1980 RDAs

Category	Group	Calories (actual)‡	Protein	Fat	Carbohydrate
Measurement Units				Grams	
Macrobiotic Menu Totals*	all	2126	79.0	40.2	361.1
U.S. RDAs†—Males	ages 23-50	2381	56.0	—	—
U.S. RDAs†—Females	ages 23-50	1565	44.0	—	—

Note: A dash means that there is no official RDA for that nutrient.

Sources:

* Estimated nutritional content of this macrobiotic menu is based on *USDA Composition of Foods Handbook No. 8.*

†The figures used were established by the U.S. Food and Drug Administration in 1980.

‡Data on American calorie intake is from *USDA Nationwide Food Comparison Survey, 1977-78,* issued by the United States Department of Agriculture.

§The average daily sodium intake among American adults is 6000–18,000 milligrams.

Calcium	Phosphorus	Iron	Sodium §	Potassium	Vitamin A	Vitamin B_1 (thiamine)	Vitamin B_2 (riboflavin)	Niacin	Vitamin C (ascorbic acid)
Milligrams					I.U.		Milligrams		
859	1539	39.3	2560	3666	14,789	3.07	1.85	20.3	236
800	800	10.0	—	—	5000	1.40	1.60	18.0	60
800	800	18.0	—	—	5000	1.00	1.20	13.0	60

Appendix B
Macrobiotic Home Remedies

Macrobiotics is concerned with keeping people well, through a wholesome diet, moderate exercise, and a balanced lifestyle. Although a balanced diet of whole foods is the best and safest path to good health, we must still be prepared for those times when the body may get out of balance. These imbalances may be due to past abuses, extreme environmental conditions, or other factors. The macrobiotic home remedies that follow are based on traditional medicines which have been used for thousands of years in many parts of the world to alleviate symptoms brought on by dietary and lifestyle imbalances. If you have any doubts about the advisability of any of these home remedies, consult an experienced macrobiotic counselor before using them. Persons with serious illness are of course advised to seek appropriate medical, nutritional, and psychological care.

Macrobiotic counselors and others who already have some familiarity with macrobiotic home remedies will find the following list to be a useful reference. For each remedy, instructions for preparation follow a brief description of the item's purposes. If you are a newcomer to macrobiotics, and you are interested in using these home remedies, consult an experienced macrobiotic counselor first.

You will notice that almost all of these home remedies are derived from macrobiotic diet foods that are discussed elsewhere in this book. This is just one aspect of the Unifying Principle, that is, the interrelatedness of all things. The foods we eat do not merely satisfy hunger; they have a profound effect upon our health as well.

Macrobiotics is the art of understanding these effects and using them to create balance and harmony.

HOME REMEDIES

Note: Use natural-material cookware when preparing medicinal drinks: glass, ceramic, or earthenware.

Bancha Stem Tea. Bancha stem tea is helpful in strengthening metabolism in the case of fatigue or illness. To prepare, use one tablespoon of tea to one quart of water. Bring tea to a boil, reduce flame, cover, and simmer for no more than five minutes. Use bancha stem tea after meals; in many cases two to three cups a day may be used.

Barley Green Tea. Barley green is the dried powder of young barley grass. It helps the body in burning up fats and eliminating toxins arising from the use of animal foods. It also helps to cleanse the liver. To prepare, place one or two teaspoons of powder in a cup. Add hot water and drink. Consult an experienced macrobiotic counselor regarding the length of use.

Brown Rice Cream.   Brown rice cream is especially helpful in cases where digestion is impaired due to a debilitating illness. To prepare, wash brown rice and then dry-roast in a skillet evenly until all the grains turn golden in color. Add three to six parts water and a little sea salt and pressure cook for two hours. Squeeze the creamy portion of the cooked rice gruel through a clean cheesecloth. Serve the rice cream with a small amount of condiment such as umeboshi plum, gomashio, tekka, kelp or kombu powder. Rice cream may be used two or more times a day, in whatever amount is desired.

Brown Rice Plaster. Brown rice plaster is used to reduce heat and swelling on an unopened boil or infection. To make the plaster, grind seven parts cooked brown rice with two parts raw green leafy vegetables (such as the outer leaves of cabbage, collards, or kale), and one part raw nori sea vegetable. Grind in a suribachi—the more the mixture is ground, the better. If it gets too sticky, add pure spring water. Apply paste to the affected area and cover with a clean cloth or towel. If plaster heats up, remove it, clean the area with warm water, and repeat if desired.

Buckwheat Plaster. Buckwheat plaster helps to draw retained water or excess fluid from tissues through the skin. It can be used effectively to reduce swelling due to water retention. To prepare, mix buckwheat flour with enough hot water to form a stiff dough. Apply a half-inch layer to the affected area and hold it in place with a clean bandage or piece of cotton linen. For either of the problems mentioned above, you may replace the plaster every four hours. A buckwheat plaster will usually reduce swelling considerably after only several applications, or at most two to three days.

Burdock Tea. Burdock tea is a tonic used for increasing overall vitality. To prepare, add a tablespoon of burdock root shavings to one cup of water. Bring to a boil, reduce flame, cover, and simmer for ten minutes.

Daikon Drinks. Three excellent drinks can be made using daikon radish (Figure B.1). The first is helpful in reducing a fever by inducing perspiration. The second can be used as a diuretic, and the third helps to dissolve excess fat and mucus in the body. To make the first drink, mix a half-cup of freshly grated daikon with a tablespoon of tamari soy sauce and one-quarter teaspoon of freshly grated ginger. Pour hot bancha tea over the mixture. Drink hot.

Figure B.1   Daikon

To make the second drink, squeeze two tablespoons of juice from grated daikon, using a clean cheesecloth. Add a pinch of sea salt and six tablespoons of water to the daikon juice, and boil. Use this mixture only once a day and never for more than three consecutive days. Do not drink the juice without first boiling it.

To make the third daikon drink, place one tablespoon of freshly grated daikon and ten drops of tamari into a cup. Pour hot water over the mixture and drink. The best time to use this drink is just before sleeping. However, do not continue to use it for more than seven days, unless advised by an experienced macrobiotic counselor.

Dandelion Root Tea. Dandelion root tea helps tone and strengthen the heart and the small intestine. To prepare, mix one tablespoon of dried dandelion root into one quart of water and bring to a boil. Reduce flame, cover, and simmer ten minutes. Consult a macrobiotic counselor regarding the use of this tea.

Dentie. Dentie has been used in the Orient for years to prevent tooth and gum problems and to stop bleeding in nosebleeds and superficial cuts and abrasions. When used regularly in place of commercial toothpaste, dentie is effective in stopping bleeding of the gums, tightening teeth, and preventing decay. Dentie powder and paste can be purchased at health food stores or made at home. To make dentie, bake a small eggplant, including the top, until it is black. Let it cool before crushing it into a powder. Mix seven parts powder with three parts sea salt. Store in a covered dry container.

Dried Daikon Leaf Skin Wash or Hip Bath. Dried daikon leaves are especially helpful in correcting skin problems and disorders of the female reproductive organs. They also work to draw excess oils and odors from the skin. Dry the leaves of several daikon radish plants in a shaded area until they turn brown and brittle. Use turnip leaves if daikon leaves are not available. The dried leaves may be stored in a covered dry container for up to a year.

To prepare, place between twenty and thirty leaves in four to five quarts of water. Bring mixture to a boil, reduce flame, cover, and simmer for fifteen minutes or until the water becomes brown. Stir in a handful of sea salt. Strain out the leaves, returning the liquid to the pot.

For skin problems, dip a clean piece of cotton or a cotton wash-cloth into the hot liquid, squeeze most of the hot liquid from it, and making sure it won't burn the skin, apply to the affected area. As the cloth cools, remove it and re-apply until the skin is quite heated. For disorders of the female reproductive organs, pour the liquid in-to a hot bath (waist level). Cover the upper body with a towel and sit in the bath for about ten minutes or until perspiration begins. Arame can also be used for the bath. Following the bath, douche with warm bancha tea with the juice of half a lemon and a pinch of sea salt added to it. Repeat as needed for up to ten days.

Ginger Compress.   The ginger compress is used to stimulate cir-culation of the blood and lymph. When applied to the skin, it helps to loosen and dissolve stagnated toxic matter, cysts, and tumors. However, in the case of cancer illness, it should be used for a short time only (five minutes maximum) as a preparation for a taro potato or buckwheat plaster. *Note:* If used as an independent treatment, the ginger compress could potentially accelerate the growth of can-cer, especially of yin types.

To prepare a ginger compress, grate a handful of ginger root (See Figure B.2) and place it in a clean cheesecloth. Squeeze the juice in-to a pot containing a gallon of hot (but not boiling) water. Do not boil the mixture. To use, dip a clean cotton towel into the ginger water and wring it out tightly, as illustrated in Figure B.3. While it is still hot, place it on the affected area. Another (dry) towel can be placed on top of the ginger compress to reduce heat loss. Apply a fresh hot towel every five to seven minutes until the skin is quite heated.

Figure B.2   Ginger Root

Figure B.3   Ginger Compress

Ginger-Sesame Oil.   Applied to the skin, ginger-sesame oil stimulates circulation by activating the function of the blood capillaries. It is also used to relieve aches and pains. To prepare, mix the juice of freshly grated ginger with an equal amount of sesame oil. To apply, dip clean cotton linen into this mixture and rub briskly onto the affected area.

Grated Raw Daikon.   Grated raw daikon is a digestive aid, especially when eaten with fatty, oily, or heavy foods, including animal products and fish. To prepare, grate a tablespoon of fresh daikon per person, and sprinkle with tamari soy sauce. Use raw red radish or raw turnip if daikon is not available.

Green Tea.   Green tea helps dissolve and discharge animal fats and excess cholesterol from the body. To make this tea, place a half-teaspoon of tea into a ceramic teapot. Pour one cup of boiling water over it and let it steep for three to five minutes. Strain and drink. Limit usage to a cupful per day. This tea is not recommended for use by individuals with an overly yin condition or illness.

Kombu Tea.   Kombu tea helps to improve blood quality and remineralize the body. To prepare, place a three-inch strip of kombu sea vegetable in a quart of water. Bring to a boil, reduce flame, cover, and simmer for ten minutes. Remove kombu and serve tea.

Kuzu (Kudzu) Tea.   Kuzu tea strengthens digestion, increases overall vitality, and reduces fatigue. To prepare, dissolve a heaping teaspoon of kuzu in a cup of cold water and stir. Bring mixture to a slight boil, reduce flame, and simmer for about five minutes, stirring occasionally. The mixture is ready when it becomes transparent. Stir in a teaspoon of tamari soy sauce and drink while still hot.

Lotus Root Plaster.   Lotus root plaster helps draw stagnated mucus from the sinuses, nose, throat and bronchi. To prepare, mix sixteen parts freshly grated lotus root (see Figure B.4) with three parts pastry flour and one part freshly grated ginger. To apply, spread a half-inch layer on a piece of cotton linen, and place the side with the lotus root directly onto the affected area. Leave the

Figure B.4   Lotus Root

plaster on for several hours or overnight. A ginger compress (page 213) can be applied before using the lotus root plaster to stimulate circulation and to loosen mucus in the affected area.

Lotus Root Tea. Lotus root tea is especially helpful in relieving coughs and dissolving mucus in the lungs. To prepare, squeeze the juice from a half-cup of freshly grated lotus root into a pot with one cup of water. Simmer until the liquid thickens, add a pinch of sea salt, and drink hot.

If fresh lotus root is unavailable, dried lotus root can be used instead. To make tea from the dried root, add two tablespoons of lotus root to one cup of water. Bring to a boil, reduce flame, and simmer for fifteen minutes. Add a pinch of sea salt or a dash of tamari, and drink hot.

Mustard Plaster. Mustard plaster is used to stimulate circulation and to loosen stagnated materials from an affected area. To prepare mustard plaster for adults, add enough hot water to dry mustard powder to make a paste. Spread this mixture onto a paper towel, cover with another, and place this "sandwich" between two thick cotton towels. Apply to the affected area and leave on until the skin becomes quite warm. Remove and wash remaining mustard from skin with warm water.

Salt Bancha Tea. Salt bancha tea is used to cleanse the body passages of stagnated matter. To prepare, add about a half-teaspoon of sea salt per cupful of warm (body temperature) bancha tea. To cleanse the nasal passageways, inhale a small amount of the mixture through one nostril at a time, and expectorate rather than swallow any that reaches the mouth. Salt bancha tea can also be used as a mouthwash to soothe a sore throat, or as a douche to cleanse the vaginal region.

Salt Pack. Salt packs can be used to warm any part of the body and to relieve muscle stiffness, aches and pains, or eliminative problems where the use of heat is desired. To prepare a salt pack, roast sea salt in a dry skillet until hot. Use enough salt to cover the affected area with a layer a half-inch thick. Wrap the hot salt in a thick cotton linen pillowcase or towel. Place a folded towel on the affected area to prevent burns, and apply salt pack. Replace the pack with another when it begins to cool.

Salt Water. A pint of water with two to four tablespoons of sea salt in it can be used either cold or hot in various ways. Cold salt water is effective in soothing irritations caused by minor burns. To use, soak the burnt area in a basin of cold salt water. Warm (body temperature) salt water is effective as an enema for relief of constipation or fat and mucus accumulation in the lower bowel. It may also be used as a douche to dissolve fat and mucus accumulations in the vagina.

Sesame Oil. Sesame oil is effective in relieving constipation. To use, mix one or two tablespoons raw sesame oil with a quarter teaspoon each of freshly grated ginger and tamari soy sauce. Take this mixture on an empty stomach.

Shiitake Mushroom Tea. Shiitake mushroom tea acts as a mild relaxant to relieve overly tense muscles and nerves. It also helps dissolve excess animal fats. To prepare, soak a dried shiitake mushroom in one cup of water for twenty minutes, then cut into quarters. Add another cup of water and simmer for twenty minutes with a pinch of sea salt. Drink only a half-cupful at a time.

Tamari Bancha Tea. Tamari bancha tea helps neutralize an overly acid blood condition. To prepare, pour one cup of bancha twig tea into a teacup and stir in two teaspoons of tamari. Drink hot.

Figure B.5 Taro Potato (Albi)   **Figure B.6 Taro Potato Plaster**

Taro Potato (Albi) Plaster. Taro potato plaster has the effect of removing toxins from the body. It is especially effective in drawing the minerals that are often contained in tumors out through the skin. When used regularly in combination with the macrobiotic diet, taro plasters will help to gradually reduce the size of tumors.

Taro potatoes can be obtained at many supermarkets and from Chinese, Armenian, Portuguese and Puerto Rican grocers. Taro are shaped like regular potatoes, with brown hair on them (see Figure B.5). Buy relatively small potatoes for use in the plaster.

In many cases it is best to apply a ginger compress (page 213) before using the taro plaster. To prepare the plaster, peel and grate enough potatoes to cover the area with a half-inch thick layer. Add one part freshly grated ginger root for every nineteen parts grated potato. Apply a half-inch-thick layer of this mixture to a piece of clean cotton linen as shown in Figure B.6. Place the side with the potato directly onto the affected area. Change every four hours. If desired, the plaster may be left on overnight without changing. If the affected area becomes cold, replace the plaster with a hot ginger compress for three minutes before placing another plaster on the area. If the chill persists, use a salt pack (see page 216) to warm the area, but do not overheat.

If taro potatoes are not available in your area, you can purchase dried taro powder and make a plaster by adding pure spring water and ginger root to it. Or you can grate an ordinary potato and mix eight parts of it with eight parts crushed (use mortar and pestle to crush) raw leafy green vegetables such as the outer leaves of cabbage, collard greens or kale, one part freshly grated ginger, and enough whole wheat flour to make a paste. While not as effective as a taro plaster, this will still produce a beneficial result.

Tofu Plaster. Tofu plaster is effective in drawing out a fever. To prepare, squeeze the water out and mash the tofu. For every six parts tofu, add one part freshly grated ginger and three parts pastry flour. Mix ingredients to make a paste and apply directly to the skin. Change plaster every two or three hours, or sooner if it becomes very hot.

Ume Extract. Ume extract is made from umeboshi plums. It is available at many health foods stores. To use, pour hot water or bancha tea over a quarter-teaspoon of the extract, and drink hot.

Umeboshi Plum. Umeboshi plums can be eaten fresh (pitted), dried and powdered, or baked. In any of these forms umeboshi helps to normalize digestion. It is especially helpful in reducing stomach acidity and in relieving temporary intestinal ailments. To use, take a half or whole plum with a cup of bancha tea. Powdered umeboshi may be taken with either hot water or bancha tea. Place a tablespoon of powdered umeboshi plum in one cup of hot water or tea, and drink hot.

Ume-Sho-Bancha. Ume-sho-bancha strengthens the blood and overall condition through normalizing digestion. To prepare, pour one cup of bancha tea over the meat of half an umeboshi plum and one teaspoon of tamari soy sauce. Stir and drink hot.

Ume-Sho-Bancha with Ginger. Like ume-sho-bancha, this tea aids digestion, and also stimulates circulation. Prepare as above, adding a quarter teaspoon of grated ginger juice to a cup of ume-sho-bancha.

Ume-Sho-Kuzu. Ume-sho-kuzu is especially helpful as a digestive aid. It also helps normalize and tone the intestines. Prepare kuzu drink according to the instructions given on page 214. Add half an umeboshi plum and one teaspoon of tamari soy sauce. One-eighth teaspoon of freshly grated ginger may also be added.

Appendix C
Glossary

The following glossary describes macrobiotic foods, cooking methods, kitchen equipment, and ideas that may not be familiar to you. Words that have particular application to the relationship between diet and health are also included.

Acupressure. A healing art based on stimulating and balancing the flow of electromagnetic energy through the meridians of the body. Acupressure utilizes finger and hand pressure on acupuncture points of the body.

Acupuncture. A Far Eastern medical technique used to re-establish balance and relieve pain by releasing blockages of energy. Acupuncture uses needles or *moxa* (a substance that is burned) placed on or in specific points along the meridians.

Aduki Beans. Small, dark red beans. Especially good when cooked with kombu. This bean may also be referred to as *adzuki* or *azuki*.

Agar-agar. A white gelatinous substance derived from a sea vegetable. Agar-agar is used in making aspics and kanten. *See also:* Kanten.

Albi. *See* Taro.

Amasake (Rice Milk). A sweetener or refreshing drink made from sweet rice and koji starter that is allowed to ferment into a thick liquid. Hot amasake is a delicious beverage on cold autumn or winter nights.

Arame. A dark brown, spaghetti-like sea vegetable similar to hijiki. Rich in iron, calcium, and other minerals, arame is often used as a side dish.

Arrowroot. A starch flour processed from the root of an American native plant. It is used as a thickening agent, similar to cornstarch or kuzu, for making sauces, stews, and desserts.

Azuki. *See* Aduki Beans.

Bancha Tea. Correctly named *kukicha*, bancha consists of the twigs and leaves from mature Japanese tea bushes. Bancha aids digestion, is high in calcium, and contains no chemical dyes. It makes an excellent breakfast or after-dinner beverage.

Barley, Pearl. A strain of barley native to China, pearl barley grows well in cold climates. It is good in stews and soups, or cooked with other grains. Pearl barley helps the body to eliminate animal fats.

Barley Malt. A thick, dark brown sweetener made from barley. Pure (100 percent) barley malt is used in making desserts, sweet and sour sauces, and in a variety of medicinal drinks.

Beefsteak Plant. *See* Shiso.

Black Sesame Seeds. Small black seeds used occasionally as a garnish or to make black gomashio, a condiment. These seeds are different from the usual white or tan variety.

Black Soybeans. *See* Japanese Black Beans.

Bok Choy. A leafy, green vegetable with thick white stems that resemble stalks. Bok choy is used mostly in summer cooking. It is sometimes called *pok choy*.

Brown Rice. Unpolished rice with only its tough outer husk removed. It comes in three main varieties: short, medium, and long grain. Short grain brown rice contains the best balance of minerals, protein, and carbohydrates, but the other types may also be used on occasion. *See also:* Sweet Brown Rice.

Brown Rice Miso. *See* Genmai Miso.

Brown Rice Vinegar. A very mild and delicate vinegar made from fermented brown rice or sweet brown rice. Brown rice vinegar is not as acid-forming in the body as apple cider vinegar.

Buckwheat. A cereal plant native to Siberia, buckwheat has been a staple food in many European countries for several centuries. It is frequently eaten in the form of kasha, whole groats, or soba noodles.

Burdock. A hardy plant that grows wild throughout the United States. The long, dark burdock root is delicious in soups, stews, and sea vegetable dishes, or sautéed with carrots. It is highly valued in macrobiotic cooking for its strengthening qualities. The Japanese name is *gobo*.

Chemical Additives. Any of the various artificial flavorings, coloring agents, or preservatives, not naturally found in foods, that are used in refining and processing. Over three thousand chemical additives have been approved by the U.S. Food and Drug Administration.

Chinese Cabbage. A large, leafy vegetable with pale green tops and thick white stems. Sometimes called *nappa*, this juicy, slightly sweet vegetable is good in soups and stews, vegetable dishes, and pickled.

Cholesterol. A compound manufactured in the human body, important in the structure of membranes and the formation of certain hormones. Cholesterol is also a constituent of all animal products. When consumed in excess in the diet, cholesterol increases the risk of gallstones, heart disease, cancer, and other health problems.

Complex Carbohydrates. Those starches, known chemically as polysaccharides, which provide the body with a high proportion of usable energy over a period of several hours. Complex carbohydrates are the major component of the macrobiotic diet. A source of energy, they are supplied primarily by whole grains, vegetables, and beans.

Condition. An individual's present state of health, rather than his or her state of health at birth, or *constitution.*

Constitution. An individual's characteristics, determined before birth by the health and vitality of his or her parents, grandparents, and other ancestors. *See also:* Condition.

Couscous. A partially refined and quick-cooking cracked wheat that has a flavor similar to cream of wheat.

Daikon. A long, white radish. Besides making a delicious side dish, daikon helps dissolve stagnant fat and mucous deposits that have accumulated in the body. Freshly grated raw daikon is especially helpful in the digestion of oily foods.

Discharge. The body's elimination of stored mucus, fat, and toxins through a variety of means, including urination, defecation, perspiration, coughing, boils, cysts, and tumors.

Do-In. A form of Oriental exercise and self-message that works to harmonize and balance the electromagnetic energy flowing through the meridians.

Dried Daikon. Daikon sold in dried and shredded form. Dried daikon is especially good cooked with kombu and seasoned with tamari soy sauce. Soaking dried daikon before use brings out its natural sweetness.

Dried Tofu. Tofu that has been naturally dehydrated by freezing. Used in soups, stews, vegetable and sea vegetable dishes, dried tofu contains less fat than regular tofu. *See also:* Tofu.

Dulse.   A reddish-purple sea vegetable used in soups, salads, and vegetable dishes. Dulse is high in protein, iron, Vitamin A, iodine, and phosphorus. Most of the dulse sold in America comes from Canada, Maine, and Massachusetts.

Electromagnetic Energy.   Energy that flows through all things, including the human body. Electromagnetic energy is generated by the earth's rotation and orbit.

Fermentation.   The action of certain bacteria or enzymes, changing the chemical composition of foods and making them easier to digest. Fermented foods on the macrobiotic diet include sauerkraut, pickles, sourdough breads, and some soyfoods.

Fiber.   The indigestible portion of whole foods; particularly, the bran of whole grains and the outer skin of legumes, vegetables, and fruits. Fiber facilitates the passage of waste through the intestines. Foods that are refined, processed, or peeled are low in fiber.

Fu.   A dried wheat gluten product. Available in thin sheets or thick round cakes, fu is a satisfying high-protein food used in soups, stews, and vegetable dishes.

Genmai Miso.   Miso made from soybeans, brown rice, and sea salt, fermented for approximately twelve months. Used in making soups and seasoning vegetable dishes. Also called *brown rice miso*.

Ginger.   A spicy, pungent, golden-colored root, used as a garnish or seasoning in cooking and for various beverages. Also used in making external home remedies such as the ginger compress.

Ginger Compress.   A hot compress, made from the juice of ginger root and water, which stimulates circulation and dissolves stagnation in the part of the body to which it is applied.

Gluten (Wheat).   The sticky substance that remains after the bran has been kneaded and rinsed from whole wheat flour. Gluten is used to make seitan and fu.

Gobo. *See* Burdock.

Gomashio. Also known as *sesame salt*. Gomashio is a table condiment made from roasted, ground sesame seeds and sea salt. It is good sprinkled on brown rice and other whole grains.

Goma Wakame Powder. A condiment made from roasted and crushed wakame and sesame seeds. Rich in minerals and other essential nutrients, goma wakame powder can be used like gomashio.

Gomoku Rice. A hearty dish traditionally made from varied combinations of four whole grains and one type of bean. Gomoku is especially good during the autumn and winter months.

Grain Coffee. A non-stimulating, caffeine-free coffee substitute made from roasted grains, beans, and roots. Ingredients are combined in different ways to create a variety of different flavors. Used like instant coffee.

Green Nori Flakes. A sea vegetable condiment made from a certain type of nori, different from the packaged variety. The flakes are rich in iron, calcium, and Vitamin A. They can be sprinkled on whole grains, vegetables, salads, and other dishes.

Hatcho Miso. Miso made from soybeans and sea salt and fermented for a minimum of two years. It has a mild salt taste and may be used from time to time in making soup stocks and condiments, and for seasoning vegetable dishes. This dark, rich miso is especially good in cold weather.

Hijiki. A dark brown sea vegetable that turns black when dried. It has a spaghetti-like consistency, a stronger taste than arame, and is very high in calcium and protein. The hijiki sold in the United States is imported from Japan or harvested off the coast of Maine.

Hokkaido Pumpkin. There are two varieties of Hokkaido pumpkin. One has a deep orange color and the other has a light green skin similar to Hubbard squash. Both varieties are very sweet and have a tough outer skin.

Hydrogenation. A process by which vegetable oils are made more saturated, causing them to become denser and more solid.

Japanese Black Beans. A special type of soybean grown in Japan. They can be used to alleviate problems of the reproductive organs. In cooking, these black beans are used in soups and side dishes.

Kampyo. Dried gourd strips which are first soaked and then used to bind vegetable rolls. The kampyo can be eaten along with the vegetable rolls.

Kanten. A jelled dessert made from agar-agar. It can include seasonal fruits such as melon, apples, berries, peaches, and pears, or amasake, aduki beans, and other items. Usually served chilled, it is a refreshing alternative to conventional gelatin.

Kasha. Buckwheat groats that are roasted prior to boiling. Kasha is a traditional Eastern European and Russian food.

Kayu. Cereal grain cooked with five to ten times as much water as grain for a long period of time. Kayu is ready when it is soft and creamy.

Kelp. A large family of sea vegetables that grow profusely off both coasts of the United States. Kelp is widely available at natural foods stores, packaged whole, granulated, or powdered. It is an excellent source of minerals, including iodine.

Kinpura. Sautéed root vegetables cut into matchsticks, usually burdock or burdock and carrots seasoned with tamari soy sauce. This hearty dish is warming and vitalizing, making it ideal for autumn and winter use.

Koji. A grain, usually semi-polished or polished rice, inoculated with bacteria and used to begin the fermentation process in a variety of foods, including miso, amasake, tamari, natto, and sake.

Kokkoh. A porridge especially for babies, made from brown rice, sweet brown rice, aduki beans, sesame seeds, and kombu. A little yinnie (rice) syrup or barley malt may be used to sweeten it.

Kombu. A wide, thick, dark green sea vegetable that is rich in minerals. Kombu is often cooked with beans and vegetables. A single piece may be re-used several times to flavor soup stocks.

Konnyaku. A gelatinous mold made in Japan from wild mountain potatoes. There are several varieties; all must be boiled and rinsed to remove their strong bitter taste before they are added to other dishes. Used in sea vegetable and nishime dishes.

Kudzu. *See* Kuzu.

Kukicha. *See* Bancha Tea.

Kuzu. A white starch made from the root of the wild kuzu plant. In this country, the plant densely populates the southern states, where it is called *kudzu*. It is used in making soups, sauces, desserts, and medicinal beverages.

Lotus. The root and seeds of a water lily that is brown-skinned with a hollow, chambered, off-white inside. Lotus is especially good for the sinuses and lungs. The seeds are used in grain, bean, and sea vegetable dishes.

Macrobiotics. An approach to balanced living, based on a balanced diet, moderate exercise, harmony with the environment, and an understanding of the philosophic principles of yin and yang. George Ohsawa was the first to recognize how these traditional concepts could be applied to modern living.

Meridian. In Oriental medicine, a pathway through which electromagnetic energy flows in the body. The healing arts acupuncture, shiatzu, and do-in, along with the martial arts, strive to re-establish harmony of the energy flow through the many meridians of the body.

Millet. A small, yellow grain that comes in many varieties, with pearled millet being the most common. Millet is used in soups, vegetable dishes, casseroles, and as a cereal.

Mirin. A cooking wine made from whole grain sweet rice. Be careful when purchasing mirin, as many varieties on the market have been processed with refined grain and additives.

Miso. A protein-rich fermented soybean paste made from ingredients such as soybeans, barley, and brown or white rice. Miso is used in soup stocks and as a seasoning. When consumed on a regular basis, it aids circulation and digestion. Mugi miso is usually best for daily use, but other varieties may be used occasionally. Quick or short-term misos, which are fermented for several weeks, are less suitable for frequent use; their salt content is higher than that of the longer-term varieties such as mugi and hatcho miso. *See also:* Genmai Miso, Hatcho Miso; Mugi Miso; Natto Miso; Onazaki Miso; Red Miso; White Miso; Yellow Miso.

Miso, Puréed. Miso that has been reduced to a smooth, creamy texture that will allow it to blend easily with other ingredients. To purée miso, place it in a bowl or suribachi and add enough water or broth to make a smooth paste. Blend with a wooden pestle or spoon.

Mochi. A heavy rice cake or dumpling made from cooked, pounded sweet brown rice. Mochi is especially good for lactating mothers, as it promotes the production of breast milk. Mochi can be prepared at home or puchased ready-made; it makes an excellent snack.

Mugicha. A tea made from roasted unhulled barley and water. Mugicha may be served hot, or as a refreshing chilled beverage in the summer.

Mucus. Secretion of mucous membranes, normally serving to protect and lubricate many parts of the body. Illness, environmental pollution, smoking, and the consumption of excess fats, sugar, and flour products can stimulate the overproduction of mucus and clog body passageways, preventing the body from expelling harmful substances.

Mugi Miso.   A miso made from barley, soybeans, and sea salt, fermented for about eighteen to twenty-four months. This flavorful miso can be used on a daily basis year-round to make soup stocks, condiments, and pickles, and to season vegetable or bean dishes. Mugi miso is generally suitable for use by individuals with serious illness.

Mu Tea.   Tea made from a blend of traditional, non-stimulating herbs. A warming and strengthening beverage, mu tea is especially beneficial for the female reproductive organs. Two popular varieties of mu tea are #9 and #16.

Nappa.   *See* Chinese Cabbage.

Natto.   Soybeans which have been cooked, mixed with beneficial enzymes, and allowed to ferment for twenty-four hours. Natto is high in easy-to-digest protein and Vitamin B_{12}.

Natto Miso.   A condiment made from soybeans, barley, kombu, and ginger; not actually a miso.

Natural Foods.   Foods that are not processed or treated with artificial additives or preservatives. Some natural foods are partially refined using traditional methods.

Nigari.   A coagulant made from sea salt, used in making tofu.

Nishime.   A method of cooking in which different combinations of vegetables, sea vegetables, or soybean products are slow-cooked with a small amount of water and tamari soy sauce. Also referred to as *waterless cooking*.

Nori.   Thin black or dark purple sheets of dried sea vegetable. Nori is often roasted over a flame until it turns green. It is used as a garnish, wrapped around rice balls in making sushi, or cooked with tamari soy sauce as a condiment. It is rich in vitamins and minerals. It is sometimes called *laver*.

Oden.   A dish in which root vegetables, sea vegetables, soybean products, and sometimes fish are simmered together for a long time. Many combinations of ingredients are used in making this excellent winter stew.

Ohagi.   Glutenous patties made from cooked, pounded sweet rice rolled in or coated with roasted and ground sesame seeds, roasted ground nuts, puréed aduki beans and raisins, etc. Frequently eaten as a dessert.

Onazaki Miso.   A miso made from white rice, soybeans, and sea salt. Lighter in color than mugi, hatcho, and genmai miso, and slightly saltier, onazaki miso has a rich flavor. It is used occasionally in making soup stocks and for seasoning vegetable dishes.

Organic Foods.   Foods grown and harvested without the use of synthetically compounded chemical fertilizers, pesticides, herbicides, and fungicides.

Physiognomy.   The art of judging an individual's state of health by viewing his or her facial and bodily characteristics.

Pok Choy.   *See* Bok Choy.

Polyunsaturated Fats.   Term used to describe the molecular structure of the fats that are present in vegetable oils and other whole foods, including fish. While polyunsaturates are more healthful than saturated fats, overconsumption may lead to elevated fatty acid (triglyceride) levels in the bloodstream.

Pressed Salad.   Very thinly sliced or shredded fresh vegetables, combined with a pickling agent such as sea salt, umeboshi, brown rice vinegar, or tamari soy sauce, and placed in a pickle press. In the pickling process, many of the enzymes and vitamins are retained while the vegetables become easier to digest.

Red Miso.   A salty-tasting short-term fermented miso, made from soybeans and sea salt. Suitable for occasional use by individuals who are in good health. Also called *aka miso*.

Refined Oil.   Salad or cooking oil that has been chemically extracted and processed to maximize yield and extend shelf life. Refining strips an oil of its color, flavor, and aroma, and reduces its nutritive value.

Rice Balls.   Rice shaped into balls or triangles, usually with a piece of umeboshi in the center, and wrapped in toasted nori or shiso leaves to completely cover. For variety, different ingredients may be used as filling or for a coating. Rice balls are good for snacks, lunches, picnics, and traveling.

Rice Syrup.   *See* Yinnie syrup.

Sake.   Japanese rice wine containing about fifteen percent alcohol, often used in cooking.

Sake Lees.   Fermented residue from making sake (rice wine), used occasionally as a seasoning in soups, stews, vegetable dishes, and pickles. Sake lees is especially good for use in winter, as it helps to generate body heat.

Sanpaku.   A Japanese term meaning "three whites." In Oriental medicine, sanpaku describes a condition of the eyes in which the iris is generally turned upwards so that white is visible beneath. This condition may be related to poor diet, and may also be a sign of ill health or misfortune.

Saturated Fats.   Term used to describe the molecular structure of most of the fats found in red meats, dairy products, and other animal foods. An excess of these in the diet contributes to heart disease and other illnesses.

Sea Salt.   Salt obtained from evaporated sea water, as opposed to rock salt mined from inland beds. Sea salt is either sun-baked or kiln-baked. High in trace minerals, it contains no sugar or chemical additives.

Sea Vegetables. Any of a variety of marine plants used as food. Sea vegetables are a prime source of vitamins, minerals, and trace elements in the macrobiotic diet.

Seitan. Wheat gluten cooked in tamari soy sauce, kombu, and water. Seitan can be made at home or purchased ready-made at many natural foods stores. It is high in protein and has a chewy texture, making it an ideal meat substitute.

Sesame Butter. A nut butter obtained by roasting and grinding brown sesame seeds until smooth and creamy. It is used like peanut butter or in salad dressings and sauces.

Shiatzu. A form of Oriental massage which releases blockages of electromagnetic energy and harmonizes energy flow through the meridians of the body.

Shiitake. Mushrooms imported dried from Japan and available freshly grown in some parts of the United States. Either type can be used to flavor soup stocks or vegetable dishes, and dried shiitake can also be used in medicinal preparations. These mushrooms help the body to discharge excess animal fats.

Shio Kombu. Pieces of kombu cooked for a long time in tamari soy sauce and used sparingly as a condiment. Shio kombu has a strong salty taste.

Shio Nori. Pieces of nori cooked for a long time in tamari soy sauce and water. Used occasionally as a condiment, shio nori makes a particularly tasty relish.

Shiso. A red, pickled leaf. The plant is known in English as the *beefsteak plant*. Shiso leaves are used to color umeboshi plums and as a condiment. Sometimes spelled *chiso*.

Shoyu. *See* Tamari and Tamari Soy Sauce.

Simple Sugars. A source of quick but short-lasting energy. Simple sugars include sucrose (table sugar), fructose, glucose (dextrose), and lactose (milk sugar). Up to fifty percent of the carbohydrates consumed in the average modern diet are simple sugars. *See also:* Complex Carbohydrates.

Soba.   Noodles made from buckwheat flour or a combination of buckwheat and (whole) wheat flour. Soba can be served in broth, in salads, or with vegetables. In the summer, soba noodles are good chilled.

Somen.   Very thin white or whole wheat Japanese noodles. Thinner than soba and other whole grain noodles, somen are often served during the summer.

Sprouted Wheat Bread.   A whole-grain bread made from soaked wheat that is sprouted and baked. Sprouted wheat bread does not contain flour, salt, or oil, and is very sweet and moist.

Suribachi.   A special serrated, glazed clay bowl. Used with a pestle, called a surikogi, for grinding and puréeing foods. An essential item in the macrobiotic kitchen, the suribachi can be used in a variety of ways to make condiments, spreads, dressings, baby foods, nut butters, and medicinal preparations.

Surikogi.   A wooden pestle that is used with a suribachi. Used to make gomashio, sea vegetable powders, and other condiments, and to mash foods to obtain a creamy consistency.

Sushi.   Rice rolled with vegetables, fish, or pickles, wrapped in nori, and sliced in rounds. Sushi is becoming increasingly popular throughout the United States. The most healthful sushi is made with brown rice and other natural ingredients.

Sushi Mat.   Very thin strips of bamboo that are fastened together with cotton thread so that they can be rolled tightly yet allow air to pass through freely. These mats are used in rolling sushi, and also to cover freshly cooked foods or leftovers.

Sweet Brown Rice.   A sweeter-tasting, more glutenous variety of brown rice. Sweet brown rice is used in mochi, ohagi, dumplings, baby foods, vinegar, and amasake. It is often used in cooking for festive occasions.

Tahini. A nut butter obained by grinding hulled white sesame seeds until smooth and creamy. It is used like sesame butter.

Takuan. Daikon which is pickled in rice bran and sea salt. It is named after the Buddhist priest who invented this particular pickling method. Sometimes spelled *takuwan*.

Tamari and Tamari Soy Sauce. Tamari soy sauce is traditional, naturally made soy sauce, as distinguished from chemically processed varieties. Original or "real" tamari is the liquid poured off during the process of making hatcho miso. The best-quality tamari soy sauce is naturally fermented for over a year and is made from whole soybeans, wheat, and sea salt. Tamari soy sauce is sometimes referred to as *shoyu*.

Taro. A type of potato with a thick, dark brown, hairy skin. It is eaten as a vegetable or used in the preparation of plasters for medicinal purposes. Also called *albi*.

Tekka. A condiment made from hatcho miso, sesame oil, burdock, lotus root, carrot, and ginger root. Tekka is sautéed over a low flame for several hours. It is dark brown in color and very rich in iron.

Tempeh. A traditional soyfood, made from split soybeans, water, and beneficial bacteria, and allowed to ferment for several hours. Tempeh is eaten in Indonesia and Sri Lanka as a staple food. Rich in easy-to-digest protein and Vitamin B_{12}, tempeh is available prepackaged in some natural foods stores.

Tempura. A method of cooking in which seasonal vegetables and fish or seafood are coated with batter and deep-fried in unrefined oil. Tempura is often served with soup and pickles.

Tofu. Soybean curd, made from soybeans and nigari. Tofu is a protein-rich soyfood used in soups, vegetable dishes, dressings, etc. *See also:* Dried Tofu.

Toxin. A poisonous compound of animal or vegetable origin which stimulates the production of antibodies.

Udon. Japanese-style noodles made from wheat, whole wheat, or whole wheat and unbleached white flour. Udon have a lighter flavor than soba (buckwheat) noodles and can be used in the same ways.

Umeboshi. Salty, pickled plums that stimulate the appetite and digestion and aid in maintaining an alkaline blood quality. Shiso leaves impart a reddish color and natural flavoring to the plums during pickling. Umeboshi can be used whole or in the form of a paste.

Umeboshi Vinegar. A salty, sour vinegar made from umeboshi plums. Diluted with water, it is used in sweet and sour sauces, salads, salad dressings, etc.

Unifying Principle. The principle of yin and yang, the philosophical foundation of macrobiotics. The Unifying Principle states that everything in the universe is constantly changing and that antagonistic forces complement one another. An understanding of this principle promotes harmony of body and mind and helps individuals to achieve balance with the natural world. *See also:* Yang; Yin.

Unrefined Oil. Pressed and/or solvent-extracted vegetable oil that retains the original color, flavor, aroma, and nutritional value of the natural substance.

Unsaturated Fats. *See* Polyunsaturated Fats.

Wakame. A long, thin, green sea vegetable used in making a variety of dishes. High in protein, iron, and magnesium, wakame has a sweet taste and delicate texture. It is especailly good in miso soup.

Wasabi. A light green Japanese horseradish that is used in sushi or traditionally with raw fish (sashimi). Wasabi is a very hot spice.

Wheat Gluten. *See* Gluten, Wheat.

Wheatberries. The grains of whole wheat are often called wheatberries. They are used to make whole wheat flours and noodles. They can also be soaked and pressure cooked with brown rice or other whole grains.

White Miso. A sweet-tasting short-term fermented miso made from white rice, soybeans, and sea salt. Used in making soup stocks and sometimes in vegetable dishes. Suitable for occasional use by individuals who are in good health. Also called *shiro miso*.

Whole Foods. The edible portions of foods as they come from nature, unprocessed, nutritionally complete, and without chemical additives. Whole foods are not refined at all.

Wild Rice. A wild grass that grows in water and is harvested by hand. Eaten traditionally by native Americans in Minnesota and other areas. These long, dark, thin grains are available at many natural foods stores.

Yang. In macrobiotics, energy or movement that has a centripetal or inward direction. One of the two antagonistic yet complementary forces that together describe all phenomena, yang is traditionally symbolized by a triangle (△). *See also:* Unifying Principle; Yin.

Yellow Miso. A short-term fermented miso made from white rice, soybeans, and sea salt. This miso has a salty but very mellow flavor and is used in making soups, sauces, and vegetable dishes. It is suitable for occasional use by individuals who are in good health.

Yin. In macrobiotics, energy or movement that has a centrifugal or outward direction and results in expansion. One of the two antagonistic yet complementary forces that together describe all phenomena, yin is traditionally symbolized by an inverted triangle (▽). *See also:* Unifying Principle; Yang.

Yinnie Syrup. A sweet, thick syrup, made from brown rice and barley, that is used in dessert cooking. This complex carbohydrate sweetener is preferable to simple sugars such as honey, maple syrup, and molasses, because the simple sugars are metabolized too quickly. Also called *rice syrup*.

Yu-Dofu. A simmered tofu and vegetable dish served in a seasoned broth. Yu-dofu is popular throughout Japan and is ideal for autumn and winter evening meals. It may be served with a variety of dips, sauces, and garnishes.

Appendix D
Transitional Foods

When you remove processed and refined food items from your shelves and cupboards, as William Dufty did, you will be taking the first step towards a more healthful lifestyle. The purpose of the chart below is to assist you in making this transition wisely and in an informed way. The chart *does not* set forth guidelines for daily eating in accordance with macrobiotic principles.

It is important to point out that while the transitional foods and ingredients listed below resemble the flavor and texture of foods that are typically part of the modern diet, and while they offer some nutritive value in place of empty calories and potentially harmful chemical additives, many of them are *suitable only for very occasional use* in macrobiotic cooking and eating.

Some of the foods and ingredients listed in the right-hand column of the chart are suggested primarily for use as replacements for the more conventional items listed on the left. They may be of use to you as transitional items during the period of time in which you are becoming familiar with macrobiotic cooking methods and techniques.

For example, if you are baking a pie, you may wish to replace the sweetener called for in your favorite recipe with barley malt, yinnie (rice) syrup, or maple syrup. You may also wish to try making the crust with arrowroot or kuzu and whole wheat pastry flour, instead of eggs and bleached white flour. In this way, you may become more sensitive to the natural flavors and qualities of your cooking ingredients. An awareness and appreciation of these properties, among others, is fundamental to the macrobiotic way. It is important to remember, however, that the use of more healthful ingredients is only one part of a more healthful lifestyle. A variety of cooking techniques and proper food combinations, as discussed throughout this book, are also important. In addition, the macrobiotic way of eating brings the body into harmony with the seasonal changes in our natural environment. The macrobiotic way of life incorporates moderate exercise and a positive philosophy as well as a healthful diet.

The recommendations about the macrobiotic way of eating are not arbitrary, but rather are founded upon the traditional ways of eating shared by many people around the world. Their efficacy has been demonstrated by the general good health and vitality, and in many cases the recovery from serious illness, of individuals who have adopted this way of eating. The standard macrobiotic dietary recommendations have been developed over many years of study and experience. In addition, trained macrobiotic counselors help individuals to modify the standard diet to suit their particular needs.

All of the dietary recommendations are based upon the proper use of whole, natural foods, and are designed to promote balance and health in the body. These qualities and strengths are needed more than ever in our complex modern world.

For information on the foods and ingredients recommended for regular use on the macrobiotic diet, see Chapters 7 and 8.

Transitional Foods

	Typical Modern Foods and Ingredients to Avoid	Transitional Foods and Ingredients (see explanation above)
Baked Goods	items made with dairy products; yeasted and refined items	home-made popcorn, rice cakes, unyeasted breads, whole grain desserts, whole grains
Beverages	alcohol, coffee, commercial caffeine and herb teas, processed fruit juices, milk, soft drinks, tap water	amasake, bancha tea, green tea, mu tea, natural fruit juices, rice wine, seed/nut milk, soymilk, spring or well water

Transitional Foods—*Continued*

Transitional Foods

	Typical Modern Foods and Ingredients to Avoid	Transitional Foods and Ingredients (see explanation above)
Fats	butter, cream, cheese, margarine, mayonnaise, milk, yogurt	nut butter; unrefined corn, olive, peanut, safflower, sesame, soy, sunflower oils
Fruits and Sweet Vegetables	canned, with preservatives, and/or sugar; dried, with additives; tropical	carrots, parsnips, squashes; natural dried fruits; temperate-climate fruits
Gelatin	all brands	agar-agar (kanten)
Proteins	beef, cheese, dark-meat fish, lamb, pork, poultry, veal	beans, seitan, soyfoods, tofu, white-meat fish, whole grains
	eggs	arrowroot or kuzu powder (used in baking), tofu
Salt	common (rock) salt, gray sea salt, iodized salt	gomashio, miso, sea salt, sea vegetable powders, tamari, tekka
Sweeteners	artificial sweeteners, chocolate, corn syrup, honey, molasses, sugar, fructose	amasake, apple juice or cider, barley malt, fresh or cooked fruits, maple syrup, mirin, natural dried fruits, yinnie (rice) syrup
White Flour Goods	all	whole wheat or other whole grain cakes, cereals, cookies, noodles, pies, etc.

Appendix E

Classes and Further Information

Further information on implementing a natural foods diet can be obtained from the East West Foundation, a nonprofit institution established in 1972. The East West Foundation and its seven major affiliates or regional offices around the country offer ongoing classes for the general public in macrobiotic cooking, Oriental medicine and philosophy, and related fields. They also provide health and dietary counseling services with trained consultants and referrals to medical doctors, registered nurses, and other professional health-care associates. Other activities include monthly weekend seminars on the macrobiotic approach to preventive health, cancer, and degenerative illness; annual summer camps in Pennsylvania and western Massachusetts; conferences and research assistance for the medical profession; and mail order books and literature. There are also Macrobiotics International and East West Centers in Canada, Mexico, Latin America, Europe, the Middle East, Africa, Asia, and Australia. The whole foods and naturally processed items described in this book are available at thousands of natural foods and health food stores, as well as a growing number of supermarkets. The macrobiotic specialty items are also available by mail order from various distributors and retailers.

Contact the one of the offices listed below for further information on any of the above educational services or to find out about the whole foods outlets in your area.

Massachusetts
Boston Headquarters:
Kushi International
P. O. Box 1100
Brookline Village, MA 02147
(617) 232-6869

Connecticut
The Macrobiotic Association
  of Connecticut
98 Washington St.
Middletown, CT 06457
(203) 344-0090

Florida
Macrobiotic Foundation of Florida
3291 Franklin Ave.
Coconut Grove, FL 33133
(305) 448-6625

Illinois
East West Center
828 Davis St.
Evanston, IL 60201
(312) 328-6632

Maryland
East West Macrobiotic
  Foundation
604 East Joppa Rd.
Towson, MD 21204
(301) 321-4474

New York
The Macrobiotic Center
  of New York
611 Broadway
New York, NY 10012
(212) 505-1010

Pennsylvania
Macrobiotic Center
243 Dickinson Street
Philadelphia, PA 19147
(215) 551-7430

For those who wish to study further, the Kushi Institute, an educational institution founded in Boston in 1979 with affiliates in London, Amsterdam, and Antwerp, offers full- and part-time instruction for individuals who wish to become macrobiotic teachers and counselors. The Kushi Institute publishes a "Macrobiotic Teachers and Counselors Directory," listing graduates who are qualified to offer guidance in the macrobiotic approach to health.

Kushi Institute
P. O. Box 7
Becket, MA 01223
(413) 623-5741

Ongoing developments in macrobiotics are reported in various publications, including the *East West Journal*, a monthly magazine begun in 1971 and now with an international readership of 200,000. The *EWJ* features regular articles on the macrobiotic approach to health and nutrition, as well as ecology, science, psychology, the arts, and pregnancy, natural birth, and child care.

> *East West Journal*
> 17 Station Street
> Brookline, MA 02147
> (617) 232-1000

Index

Healthy Habits
are easy to come by—
If You Know Where to Look!

To get the latest information on:
- better health • diet & weight loss
- the latest nutritional supplements
- herbal healing & homeopathy and more

COMPLETE AND RETURN THIS CARD RIGHT AWAY!

Where did you purchase this book?

❑ bookstore ❑ health food store ❑ pharmacy
❑ supermarket ❑ other (please specify)_____

Name _____

Street Address _____

City _____ State _____ Zip _____

Trying to eat healthier? Looking to lose weight? Frustrated with bland-tasting fat-free foods?

For more information on how you can create low-fat meals that are packed with taste and nutrition and develop healthy habits that can improve the quality of your life,

COMPLETE AND RETURN THIS CARD!

Where did you purchase this book?

❑ bookstore ❑ health food store ❑ pharmacy
❑ supermarket ❑ other (please specify)_____

Name _____

Street Address _____

City _____ State _____ Zip _____

AVERY PUBLISHING GROUP

120 Old Broadway

Garden City Park, NY 11040

AVERY PUBLISHING GROUP

120 Old Broadway

Garden City Park, NY 11040